Neurovascular Examination

Neurovascular Examination

The Rapid Evaluation of Stroke Patients Using Ultrasound Waveform Interpretation

Andrei V. Alexandrov, MD

Professor and Director
Comprehensive Stroke Center
University of Alabama at Birmingham
University of Alabama Hospital
Birmingham, AL
USA

FOREWORD BY DAVID S. LIEBESKIND

WILEY Blackwell

This edition first published 2013; © 2013 by Andrei V. Alexandrov

Blackwell Publishing was acquired by John Wiley & Sons in February 2007. Blackwell's publishing program has been merged with Wiley's global Scientific, Technical and Medical business to form Wiley-Blackwell.

Registered office: John Wiley & Sons, Ltd, The Atrium, Southern Gate, Chichester, West Sussex, PO19 8SQ, UK

Editorial offices: 9600 Garsington Road, Oxford, OX4 2DQ, UK

The Atrium, Southern Gate, Chichester, West Sussex, PO19 8SQ, UK

111 River Street, Hoboken, NJ 07030-5774, USA

For details of our global editorial offices, for customer services and for information about how to apply for permission to reuse the copyright material in this book please see our website at www.wiley.com/wiley-blackwell

Library of Congress Cataloging-in-Publication Data is available for this title

A catalogue record for this book is available from the British Library.

Wiley also publishes its books in a variety of electronic formats. Some content that appears in print may not be available in electronic books.

Cover images courtesy of the author
Cover design by Grounded Design

Set in 8.75/12 pt Meridien by Toppan Best-set Premedia Limited, Hong Kong
Printed and bound in Singapore by Markono Print Media Pte Ltd

1   2013

Contents

Foreword

The practice of stroke medicine is more than a profession that I share with Andrei, as we both indulge in this passionate hobby that extends far beyond a typical job. Andrei authored this innovative book based on his diverse background in the medical physics and technical aspects of ultrasonography, neurovascular expertise, and perpetual education of trainees to develop new treatments for acute ischemic stroke. Fueled by similar interests in engineering, neuroimaging, and mentorship of young investigators, I have pursued a collateral pathway to study the hemodynamics of cerebrovascular disorders. These multidisciplinary roots have driven us to the frontiers of our field, where questions abound regarding the use of imaging to improve treatment and the subsequent outcomes of our patients at risk of devastating stroke syndromes. We continually ask questions about the whys of stroke, seeking explanations for the complex pathophysiology of ischemia in the brain. We think about blood flow without fear of mathematics or the challenge of uncharted territory in the crevasse between various fields. In fact, we both think about flow in the snow while enjoying a similar enthusiasm for skiing every winter! On such occasions, we exchange text messages about specific hemodynamic advances intermixed with scenes of powder on the slopes. Off the slopes, we both capitalize on the wealth of imaging data provided by a diverse range of technology, from ultrasonography to multimodal CT/MRI and conventional angiography. Detailed analyses of such vast imaging datasets in the light of clinical manifestations have been the focus of intense research efforts by our collaborative groups to understand collateral circulation and reperfusion. Our shared research interests have centered on the pathophysiology and clinical relevance of serial imaging for hemodynamics in the brain rather than the development of an iso-

lated diagnostic technique or elusive treatment for stroke. In my work on collateral perfusion in acute stroke or chronic disorders of intracranial atherosclerosis and moyamoya, difficult questions arise about hemodynamics where the answers cannot be found in the literature or textbooks. At those times, I call upon Andrei to provide expertise and clarify the boundaries of known from unknown. Many other colleagues in the field have similarly suggested calling Andrei when questions arise about blood flow in stroke. This book is indeed an explanation of hemodynamic assessment with ultrasonography as best described only by Andrei.

Unlike the traditional medicine textbook where dogma is recapitulated from generation to the next, this book emphasizes process over boundless tomes of medical facts. This unique book provides the perspective and an experienced approach for burgeoning stroke professionals to utilize ultrasound at the bedside. Readers may then similarly engage in this fascinating and rewarding process where imaging technology can be integrated with neurological expertise to improve stroke treatment outcomes. After reading the book more than two times, I can attest that it will easily become an essential companion guide to this rapidly evolving field. The book covers a broad range of topics from the applied principles of ultrasound physics and related hemodynamics to clinical applications, composed in an inviting style of writing that can be easily digested. The content should be of interest to anyone exploring hemodynamics of the brain, as an introductory book or even as a refresher text for experienced researchers. The personal nature of each chapter and close integration with germane clinical issues reflects a progressive approach to stroke. Andrei notes that management of the stroke patient and treatment decisions do not end with delivery of the tPA bolus, as this is just an initial step. Decision-making may be tailored to specific aspects of a given case rather than blind adherence to standard protocols. Throughout the book, functional significance or hemodynamic effects of vascular lesions are emphasized, in sharp contrast to the overly simplistic anatomical definitions for luminal stenosis utilized to date. Neurovascular examination with ultrasonography is touted for the ability to discern key physiological details beyond limited anatomical characterization of other neuroimaging modalities. This education in plumbing for neuroscientists offers hemodynamic perspective on the role of collaterals, microcirculation and even venous phenomena. These entities and the physics of flow are described in conceptual format, allowing the reader to grasp essential concepts rather than memorizing equations. This straightforward explanation of the underlying physics sets the stage for the ultimate how-to book on cerebrovascular ultrasound while considering the limitations of current technology. A palpable interest in educating future strokologists about influential mechanisms and pathophysiology is evident throughout the book. For instance, a thoughtful discussion of intracranial stenosis and downstream blood flow is offered in place of the usual fixation solely on measures of vessel narrowing. Hemodynamics gleaned from real-time neurovascular examination and serial monitoring in parallel with clinical evaluation are emphasized, casting stroke as a dynamic process incompletely captured by static imaging studies such as the routine noncontrast CT examination inevitably described as "unremarkable".

If you believe blood flow plays an important role in determining stroke risk and subsequent outcomes, then this book on ultrasound and hemodynamics in clinical practice is undoubtedly useful. Andrei's stepwise overview on the topic in logical sequence from the requisite physics concepts to common hemodynamic scenarios will be of value in routine stroke care. The only missing aspect is an audio clip of Andrei's whistling and other vocalizations of ultrasonography findings. The hemodynamic aspects of ischemic stroke underscored in this book form the basis for next steps in stroke therapy, extending even beyond my own obvious bias on collateral perfusion!

David S. Liebeskind, MD
Professor of Neurology
Neurology Director, Stroke Imaging
Co-Director, UCLA Cerebral Blood Flow Laboratory
Program Director, Stroke and
Vascular Neurology Residency
Associate Neurology Director, UCLA Stroke Center
Los Angeles, CA, USA

Preface

The modern term stroke has a predecessor, a Greek word "apoplexy," or "striking away," as if a person was struck by the hand of God. Although some strokes are truly unexpected and unpredictable, the risk factors for most are now largely known, often detectable and some modifiable, and they tell us: stroke is coming, it could be imminent, and one has to take care and change what can be changed to prevent it.

Stroke may still happen. This misfortune has been a stepchild of medicine as it caused no pain, was thought to affect mostly the elderly, leaving a person miserably disabled, and there was nothing that a clinician could do to reverse it. Reperfusion therapy changed that, though some nihilism and resistance still linger. For those knowing how much needs to be done, there is a constant challenge to advance our ability to detect stroke, bring victims to treatment, tailor rescue to the specific mechanism of injury, and, most importantly, find ways to preserve the brain tissue and afford time for natural or induced mechanisms to heal, restore, and to protect the person's ability to get through a stroke.

What came next is our understanding that stroke is not a striking lightening rod, leaving irreversible damage. It is rather a process that takes time. Some complete the damage in minutes, some in hours, some linger for days at the edge of potential reversibility. For how long, why, and how to afford time to bring them back will be the challenge for generations of strokologists to come.

There is never an end to an exploration in science, and the time to challenge established dogmas is always now. New questions and discoveries lead to new thinking. Thinking outside the box generates unorthodox ideas. These ideas lead to innovation, disruption, and ultimately improvement in medicine. Stroke is one area that deserves this now. With so many social,

organizational issues, and truly multifactorial mechanisms, stroke poses a great challenge not only to my colleagues in Vascular Neurology, Neuro-Endovascular Specialties, Neuro-Critical Care and Emergency Medicine but to many other disciplines of science as well as health-care providers, administrators, and politicians.

Historically, stroke was seen as a neurologists' domain to "diagnose and adios" when a traditional neurological examination was used to pinpoint the location of a lesion while therapeutic options until recent times were nil, leaving physicians pessimistic. Novel developments in stroke treatment modify our classic approach to diagnostic evaluation of acute stroke victims. Often, there is no time to conduct a full neurological examination in the emergency room. Structured and focused scales are predictive of consequences of cerebrovascular catastrophes but provide little clues as to the mechanism of a specific event. Physicians taking care of stroke patients need to understand hemodynamic phenomena and applied physics of imaging. This book is a reflection of many years of emergent evaluations of stroke patients whereby my to-the-point neurological examination and treatment decision-making were complemented by bedside assessment of cerebral vasculature and hemodynamics in real time with ultrasound. The sequence of chapters reflect the areas that physicians, sonographers, and trainees need to study in order to build knowledge and skills for practicing, interpreting, and integrating cerebrovascular ultrasound for stroke patient assessment and treatment.

I have to explain how I got there myself. In the past, most neurologists were reluctant to take on stroke since it bordered so much on the internal medicine and more recently on critical care and surgery – all areas that many neurologists shied away from for a variety of reasons. I myself was no exception. I was graduating from a neurology residency with no interest in caring for a disease for which nothing radical could be done at that time (a disclosure here, it was prior to the NINDS rt-PA Stroke Study). Like cancer, like incurable diseases before actual discoveries that changed the dogmas and stigmas around these conditions, I was under the impression that what I can do as a physician will be better practiced elsewhere. I have to give credit to the director of our academic institute back in the Soviet-era Moscow, late Professor Nicolai Victorovich Vereshchagin, who told me that I had to do a stroke fellowship under Professor Dmitri Kuzmitch Lunev, whom I worshiped during my residency training (yet I was reluctant to consider stroke as my future subspecialty). It was an order, I had to obey it. Reluctantly, I did.

My subsequent journey introduced me to amazing teachers and thinkers including John W. Norris, Sandra E. Black, Patrick M. Pullicino, and ultimately to James C. Grotta, all of whom contributed to my mentoring and leading me to learning real-time pathophysiology of stroke through the prism of ultrasound, which I share with you in this book.

Andrei V. Alexandrov

Acknowledgment

This book would have never been possible to write without many hours of teaching fellows at the bedside, in emergency rooms, intensive care units, cath labs and occasionally in late night diners over "code G-man" or "code oysters" as well as setting up research projects or while reviewing and dissecting countless ultrasound waveforms and images. This book is therefore dedicated to all of them, listed in chronological order from my first trainee back in 1997 in Texas (bottom) to current fellows (top) as of 2012 at the University of Alabama at Birmingham:

Clinical Fellows in Vascular Neurology at UAB

Michael Lyerly, MD	USA
Kara Sands, MD	USA
Karen Albright, DO, MPH	USA
Luis Cava, MD	USA
Asad Chaudhary, MD	USA
Aaron Anderson, MD	USA

Clinical Stroke Fellows trained and certified in Neurosonology at UT-Houston

Andrew Barreto, MD	USA
Ken Uchino, MD	USA
Lise Labiche, MD	USA
Nicholas Okon, DO	USA
Scott Burgin, MD	USA
Robert Felberg, MD	USA
Andrew Demchuk, MD	Canada

Fellows in Cerebrovascular Ultrasound and Stroke Research (UAB, Barrow Neurological Institute and UT-Houston)

Yuri Yakov, MD	USA
Reza Bavarsad Shahripour, MD	Iran
Danny Tkatch, MSc, RVT	USA

Andrey Samal, MD	USA
Stanislava Kolieskova, MD	Slovakia
Kristian Barlinn, MD	Germany
Paola Palazzo, MD	Italy
Clotilde Balucani, MD	Italy
Yi Zhang, MD	USA
Marta Rubiera, MD	Spain
Nguen Thang, MD	Vietnam
Limin Zhao, MD	China
Georgios Tsivgoulis, MD	Greece
Vijay Sharma, MD	Singapore
Annabelle Lao, MD	Philippines
Robert Mikulik, MD	Czech Republic
Yosik Kim, MD	Korea
Yasuyuki Iguchi, MD	Japan
Chin-I Chen, MD	Taiwan
Alejandro Brunser, MD	Chile
Yong-Seok Lee, MD	Korea
Sergio Calleja, MD	Spain
Zsolt Garami, MD	Hungary
Oleg Chernyshev, MD, PhD	Russia
Ashraf El-Mitwalli, MD	Egypt
Ioannis Christou, MD	Greece

Finally, I'm blessed by an amazing relationship with my wife, Anne Alexandrov who holds a PhD in hemodynamics and who is also a clinical nurse specialist and a scientist focused on stroke. Our constant debates and her broad knowledge of emergency medicine, cardiovascular diseases, and outcomes research made me a better Vascular Neurologist. To conquer stroke, one must build a multidisciplinary team and appreciate the value each health professional brings to it. This book provides you with information that is largely underutilized by stroke specialists in the USA, while practices of ultrasound vary greatly worldwide. I hope that an alternative to what is largely becoming snap-shot imaging-based stroke care will aid clinicians with real-time assessment tools.

Abbreviations

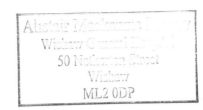

ABI	ankle–brachial index		**CVA**	cerebrovascular accident
ACA	anterior cerebral artery		**CVP**	central venous pressure
AComA	anterior communicating artery		**CW**	continuous wave
ADC	apparent diffusion coefficient		**DWI**	diffusion weighted imaging
AFib	atrial fibrillation		**EBR**	embolus-to-blood ratios
AI	acceleration index		**ECA**	external carotid artery
AIUM	American Institute of Ultrasound in Medicine		**ECASS**	European Cooperative Acute Stroke Study
ALARA	as low as reasonably achievable		**ECG**	electrocardiogram
AR	axial resolution		**ECP**	external counter-pulsation
ASPECTS	Alberta Stroke Program Emergent Computed Tomography Score		**EDV**	end diastolic velocity
			ES	embolic signal
AT	acceleration time		**FDA**	Federal Drug Administration
AVM	arteriovenous malformation		**FFT**	fast Fourier transformation
BA	basilar artery		**FLAIR**	fluid-attenuated inversion recovery
BHI	breath-holding index		**FRS**	Framingham Risk Score
BP	blood pressure		**GCS**	Glasgow Coma Scale
BPAP	bilevel positive airway pressure		**HIFU**	high-intensity focused ultrasound
B-mode	brightness modulated		**HITS**	high-intensity transient signals
BSA	body surface area		**IABP**	intra-aortic balloon pump
CABG	coronary artery bypass graft		**IAD**	intracranial atherosclerotic disease
CAS	carotid artery stenting		**ICA**	internal carotid artery
CBF	cerebral blood flow		**ICH**	intracerebral hemorrhage
CCA	common carotid artery		**ICP**	intracranial pressures
CEA	carotid endarterectomy		**IMS**	Interventional Management of Stroke trial
CHF	congestive heart failure			
CI	cardiac index		**IMT**	intima-media thickness
CLOTBUST	Combined Lysis of Thrombus in Brain Ischemia using Transcranial Ultrasound and Systemic tPA		**IRB**	Institutional Review Board
			LDL	low-density lipoprotein
			LMCA	left middle cerebral artery
CO	cardiac output		**LVAD**	left ventricular assist device
CPAP	continuous positive airway pressure		**MADV**	mean average diastolic velocity
CPP	cerebral perfusion pressure		**MAP**	mean arterial pressure
CSF	cerebrospinal fluid		**MCA**	middle cerebral artery
CT	computed tomography		**MES**	microembolic signals
CTA	computed tomography angiography		**MFV**	mean flow velocity
CTP	computed tomography perfusion		**MI**	mechanical index

MRA	magnetic resonance angiography	SPTA	spatial peak temporal average
MRI	magnetic resonance imaging	SRU	Society of Radiologists in Ultrasound
MTT	mean transit time	SV	stroke volume
MVP	mean venous pressure	SVR	systemic vascular resistance
NASCET	North American Symptomatic Carotid Endarterectomy Trial	TAMV	temporal average mean flow velocity
		TAPV	temporal average peak velocity
NIHSS	National Institutes of Health Stroke Scale	TCCS	transcranial color coded duplex sonography
NINDS	National Institutes of Neurological Disorders and Stroke	TCD	transcranial Doppler
		TEE	transesophageal echocardiography
OA	ophthalmic artery	TI	thermal index
OSA	obstructive sleep apnea	TIA	transient ischemic attack
PAVM	pulmonary arteriovenous malformation	TIB	thermal index bones
PComA	posterior communicating artery	TIBI	Thrombolysis in Brain Ischemia flow grading system
PFO	patent foramen ovale		
PI	pulsatility index	TIC	thermal index cranial bone
PICA	posterior inferior cerebellar artery	TICA	terminal internal carotid artery
PMD	power motion Doppler	TIMI	Thrombolysis in Myocardial Infarction flow grading system
PRF	pulse repetition frequency		
PSV	peak systolic velocity		
PW	pulsed wave	TIS	thermal index soft tissues
RAP	right atrial pressure	TP	transverse process
Re	Reynolds number	tPA	tissue plasminogen activator
RI	resistance index	TTE	transthoracic echocardiography
RMCA	right middle cerebral artery	TTP	time to peak
SA	sinoatrial node	tVA	terminal vertebral artery
SAH	subarachnoid hemorrhage	VA	vertebral artery
sICH	symptomatic intracerebral hemorrhage	VISTA	Virtual International Stroke Trials Archive
SM	steal magnitude	VMR	vasomotor reactivity

1 Understanding the Mechanisms and Dynamics of Cerebrovascular Events

"What does the term CVA "really" stand for? . . . Confused Vascular Assessment!"

Strokology 101

The time-honored use of a nonspecific term, CVA (cerebrovascular accident), by many of our colleagues underscores the need for patients suspected of having a stroke or a transient ischemic attack (TIA) to be seen by vascular neurologists to determine why these events are happening. This, in turn, will yield answers to the questions of how to treat and prevent stroke.

Our ability to diagnose the type of stroke (ischemic or hemorrhagic) relies solely on imaging, and patients with new symptoms suggestive of stroke should be granted emergency access to computed tomography (CT) and magnetic resonance imaging (MRI), depending on the clinical situation and resources available. Often both of these tests are done in sequence during their hospital stay or during observation/ outpatient diagnostic workup. Patients with stroke or TIA should also undergo several other tests. The reason is not only to see the parenchymal damage, if any, and tissue at risk of infarction but also to determine the pathogenic mechanism of the event because treatment options vary greatly (Figure 1.1). The focus of this book is the assessment of a stroke patient, linking the neurological findings with the evaluation of vessels, and, in turn, integrating these findings with parenchymal and perfusion imaging. This book will further explain how to obtain this information at the bedside, and how it can change patient management.

Lessons learned from cardiology and vascular medicine are invaluable for vascular neurology; however, these can only be applied to the brain vasculature to a certain extent. Unlike coronary vessels, the intracranial arteries are paper thin and cannot withstand too much mechanical or polypharmacological manipulations. They respond by vasodilation to a drop in blood pressure or volume in an attempt to maintain cerebral blood flow (CBF) as they also assure continuous diastolic flow, a feature of the low-resistance parenchymatous organs. When a patient develops stroke symptoms, this indicates that the blood flow to a specific area of the brain has dropped below the level that normally sustains neuronal function. Electrical function of neurons becomes affected at CBF falling below approximately 20 mL/100 g of brain tissue/min (Figure 1.2)[1–4]. Flattening of the electroencephalogram was seen in human subjects during endarterectomy when CBF was ≤19 mL/min [2]. The concept of ischemic penumbra emerged from studies correlating the neuronal electrical activity and CBF reduction thresholds [5]. It became clear that at certain CBF levels the neurons can remain structurally intact but functionally inactive. Without reperfusion treatment a further fall in CBF occurs, and the ischemic cascade may progress fast leading to influx of calcium and brain death. Further experimental research has focused on tissue viability thresholds [6, 7].

The neurological symptom onset has been long equated with the timing of a thromboembolic occlusion. In reality, this is not correct [8]. Symptom onset is the time of the collateral or residual flow failure. This failure can occur shortly after an acute occlusion or it can develop over time. Furthermore, the time lapse between symptom onset and initiation of reperfusion therapy was further treated as a substitute for recoverability. In general, this time dependency is applicable to large groups of patients in clinical trials: patients' chances to recover completely double

Neurovascular Examination: The Rapid Evaluation of Stroke Patients Using Ultrasound Waveform Interpretation, First Edition.
Andrei V. Alexandrov.

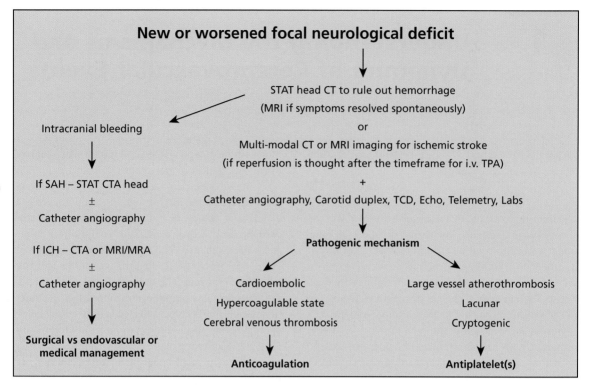

Figure 1.1 An overview of common sequences in the diagnostic workup and treatment options according to a specific pathogenic mechanism.

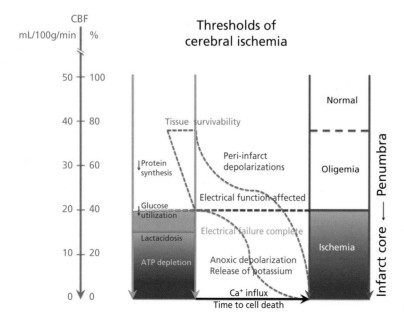

Figure 1.2 Neuronal dysfunction and levels of cerebral blood flow impairment. Two important concepts related to cerebral ischemia are schematically presented here. The decreasing levels of cerebral blood flow (CBF) due to occlusion or hypoperfusion can induce an oligemic state, subsequent electric cell dysfunction and failure, finally leading to cell death at very low CBF levels [1]. These thresholds of ischemia are hypothetically combined with the time to cell death and recoverability of tissue (dotted S-shape lines invoked from observations in reference [6]. The concepts arise from landmark studies of Austrup et al. [1] and Jones et al. [6].

Table 1.1 Main pathogenic types of ischemic stroke, or TOAST classification

Large-vessel atheromatous
≥50% stenosis or occlusion with pre-existing atheromatous plaque in an artery feeding the territory of cerebral ischemia

Cardioembolic
Identification of a known risk factor or source for cerebral embolization from the heart, i.e. atrial fibrillation, intracardiac thrombus, etc.

Lacunar
A typical lesion affecting perforating vessels in subcortical areas or pons/ brainstem

Other
Arterial dissection, paradoxical embolism, hypercoagulable state, vasculitis, etc.

Cryptogenic
No pathogenic mechanism was identified upon adequate workup or two or more etiologies were found, i.e. cortical lesion unilateral to a severe carotid stenosis in a patient with known atrial fibrillation

Data from Adams *et al.* [10].

if fibrinolytic treatment with intravenous tissue plasminogen activator (tPA) starts at 2 hours from symptom onset, and these chances diminish rapidly over time [9]. The decision making for systemic tPA is fairly straight forward and within the first few hours it applies to the majority of patients regardless of the cause of cerebral ischemia. However, a closer look at an individual patient reveals that ischemic stroke is remarkably heterogeneous (Table 1.1). We will examine in turn different stroke types and what tests are suitable to ascertain these mechanisms, commonly referred to as the TOAST classification of stroke pathogenic mechanisms [10]. Stroke remains an extremely time-sensitive process and if therapeutic attempts to restore blood flow are not done in time, most patients will loose their battles with obstructive arterial lesions. Traditional time frames for reperfusion, however, have nothing to do with the severity of ischemia and its variable mechanisms. The question is what else besides systemic tPA can you offer as treatment? This depends on why stroke is happening, and this in turn leads to the choice of imaging modalities. Even the use of systemic thrombolytics could be better gauged by rapid multimodal imaging [8, 11]. The stress here must be on "rapid," that is within minutes not half an hour to an hour to acquire imaging sequences.

Our ability to understand stroke by imaging the brain with X rays and MRI is constantly evolving, and the majority of current and future stroke specialists spend a great deal of time learning how to base their decisions on multimodal CT or MRI imaging. They also become familiar with carotid duplex ultrasound, at least to order it as a screening test for carotid pathology of the neck. Far fewer take the time and effort to master ultrasound tests themselves, particularly transcranial Doppler (TCD). In my practice, I use all available tests when appropriate or feasible, as they provide complimentary information. Furthermore, I find reasons to treat (not excuses to withhold treatment), an approach opposite to minimalistic or nihilistic views as to what we can offer stroke patients. The latter results in under-utilizing imaging and vascular assessment, often resulting in patient receiving treatment that is not based on a pathogenic mechanism specific to their event.

The following case scenarios will show how we approach typical patient problems, what key questions we ask to begin patient management, and the complimentary use of diverse ultrasound tests for the neurological examination and the standard of care CT or MRI scanning. A brief case presentation is followed by questions and answers that illustrate the thought process and supportive facts. So, as we say at the beginning of stroke rotation, welcome to the (neurovascular) plumbing service!

Case study 1.1

A 62-year-old man, current smoker with otherwise unremarkable past medical history and no primary care doctor, is seen for an episode of weakness in the left arm that lasted for 10 min and resolved spontaneously. The National Institutes of Health Stroke Scale (NIHSS) score (Appendix 1.1) is 0. A noncontrast head CT done within 20 min of arrival to the hospital is normal. His BP is 153/70 mmHg, pulse regular. ABCD^2 score (Tables 1.2 and 1.3) = 3 points [12].

Table 1.2 ABCD^2 score

Factor	Score
Age: ≥60 years	1
Blood pressure: ≥140/90 mmHg	1
Clinical features:	
Unilateral weakness	2
Speech impairment without weakness	1
Duration:	
≥60 min	2
10–59 min	1
Diabetes: Yes	1

Table 1.3 Stroke risk within 2 days after TIA as predicted by the total ABCD^2 score

Risk	ABCD^2 score (%)
Low	0–3 (1.0)
Medium	4–5 (4.1)
High	6–7 (8.1)

The ABCD^2 score is predictive of the risk of stroke after TIA and is being used to stratify patients according to this risk [12]. However, it bears no information as to pathogenic mechanism of the TIA, and it has certain other limitations. It should not be used instead of multimodal imaging such as MRI because our definition of the TIA is based on imaging of the brain parenchyma and noncontrast CT scan is not sensitive to stroke for several hours after symptom onset, particularly with spontaneous early symptom resolution.

Box 1.1 Current definition of TIA

Transient ischemic attack (TIA): a transient episode of neurological dysfunction caused by focal brain, spinal cord, or retinal ischemia, without acute infarction.

Disclaimer: The definition of TIA proposed above is not constrained by limitations of DWI or any other imaging modality. The definition is tissue based, similar to the diagnoses of cancer and myocardial infarction. However, unlike the situation with cancer but similar to that with myocardial infarction, the histological diagnosis of brain infarction typically must be inferred from clinical, laboratory, and imaging data. The most appropriate clinical, laboratory, and imaging modalities to support the diagnosis of TIA versus stroke will evolve over time as diagnostic techniques advance. Specific criteria for the diagnosis of brain infarction also will evolve, just as the laboratory criteria for the diagnosis of myocardial infarction evolved as new serum markers were identified. However, the definition of the entity will not vary; ischemic stroke requires infarction, whereas TIA is defined by symptomatic ischemia with no evidence of infarction [13].

1. What is the diagnosis?

Likely a TIA (definition provided in Box 1.1[13]).

2. What is the highest yield test that should be done next?

Multimodal head MRI with head and neck magnetic resonance angiography (MRA).

3. When should this test should be done?

As soon as possible, because TIA is a medical emergency and patients with TIA are at risk of developing a stroke. MRI/MRA in combination with the ABCD^2 score can identify those at particularly high risk of both stroke (31%) and functional impairment (23%) within 90 days [14]. Furthermore, the diagnosis of TIA versus stroke depends on our evolving imaging ability to visualize brain tissue damage [13], and a noncontrast head CT has a low yield in patients with deficits that lasted just a few minutes as opposed to many hours.

4. What information can MRI/MRA provide?

If the diffusion weighted imaging (DWI) is negative, this would confirm the diagnosis of a TIA (but will

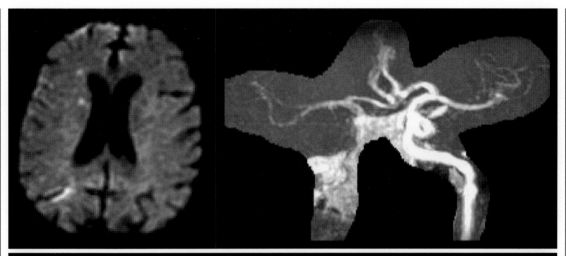

Abnormal DWI + obstruction on MRA = Stroke risk >30%
Most events "front-loaded" in next 48 h

Figure 1.3 Clinical value of MRI/MRA in estimating stroke risk after TIA. Diffusion weighted imaging (DWI) showed a small ischemic lesion in the right hemisphere/watershed distribution between the middle and anterior cerebral arteries; magnetic resonance angiography (MRA) showed an obstruction extending from the proximal right internal carotid artery.

not completely rule out a small stroke or a stroke in the posterior circulation; see further explanation in Box 1.1). If MRA is abnormal, that is it may be showing persisting arterial obstruction, this would point to a high risk of stroke symptom recurrence. Also, brain perfusion sequences on MRI can identify patients with hypoperfusion even if the DWI is negative, and this finding should raise concern for possible neurological deterioration if cerebral hemodynamics is not improved.

If DWI is positive, that is showing a lesion in the appropriate distribution with corresponding changes on the apparent diffusion coefficient (ADC) sequence and the T2 shine-through artifact is ruled out, the patient has an ischemic stroke. Abnormal DWI and abnormal MRA findings identify patients with spontaneously resolved symptoms who are at the highest risk of stroke recurrence that is "front loaded" in the next couple of days (Figure 1.3)[15].

5. What is the impact of MRI/MRA on patient management?

MRI/MRA provide the initial ascertainment of the pathogenic mechanism of the current event for early initiation of an appropriate secondary stroke prevention, and can help determine the need for admission of the patient to the hospital (demonstration of an ischemic stroke despite symptom resolution and the high risk for early recurrence). CT-angiography/ CT-perfusion (CTA/CTP) and neurovascular ultrasound tests should also be considered if patients have contraindications for MRI.

6. What is the likely pathogenic mechanism for this event?

In Caucasian patients of this age group who are smokers, atheromatous stenosis of the proximal internal carotid artery should be ruled out first [16]. Atheromatous disease in the intracranial vessels should, in the first place, be suspected in African Americans, Asians, or Hispanics but also not entirely discounted in Caucasians [16–18]. MRA may show an abnormality in these vessels but it tends to overestimate the degree of the stenosis. An absent vessel segment on MRA may not necessarily be occluded, that is this false-positive finding ("flow gap" on MRA) may occur in the setting of near-occlusion with tenuous residual flow or flow reversal due to

(*Continued*)

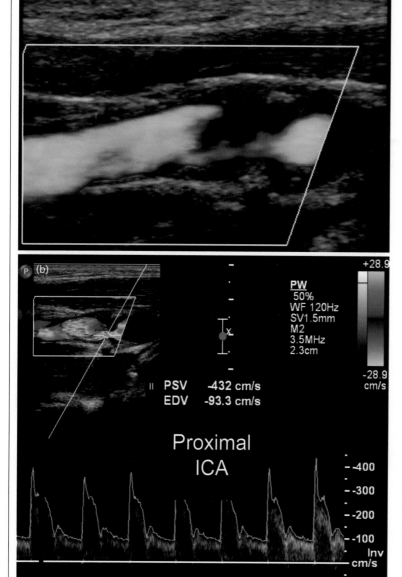

Figure 1.4 Carotid duplex findings with severe ICA atheromatous stenosis. Longitudinal views of the proximal ICA (left side of the image is oriented cephalad) show mostly hypoechoic atherosclerotic plaque and the residual lumen on power mode (**a**) and color flow (**b**). Angle-corrected velocity measurements are shown in (**b**) (PSV, peak systolic velocity; EDV, end diastolic velocity).

collateralization or in the presence of turbulence. This is why ultrasound examination of the precerebral and intracranial vessels should be done whether or not MRA shows a lesion. Looking just at reconstructed MRA images may also lead to false-negative results.

Ultrasound may show an atherosclerotic plaque (Figure 1.4), facilitating the diagnosis of atherosclerosis. This, in turn, will further support initiation of statin and antiplatelet therapy. Alternatively, ultrasound may show a thrombus without pre-existing atheroma (Figure 1.5), and this finding should prompt the search for an embolic source or a hypercoagulable state.

Ultrasound may show the presence of a ≥50% diameter reducing atheromatous stenosis in the vessel feeding the affected side of the brain (Figure 1.4). This finding will help identify patients with a large-vessel atheromatous mechanism of the event

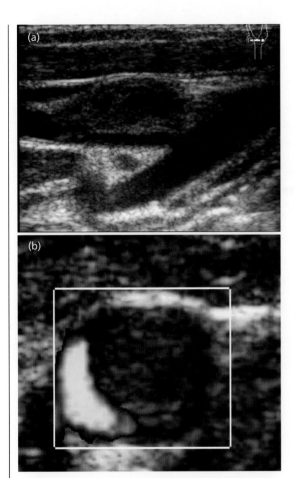

Figure 1.5 Carotid duplex visualization of a thrombus in the proximal ICA without underlying atheromatous stenosis. (**a**) Longitudinal brightness-modulated (B-mode) view of a large thrombus that is attached to the near wall occupying most of the carotid bulb. (**b**) Transverse view of the same thrombus with crescent moon-like appearance of the residual lumen on power Doppler.

(Table 1.1) and raise questions about further angiographic imaging to plan carotid revascularization for secondary stroke prevention. In fact, Figure 1.4 shows a lesion predictive of a ≥70% stenosis, according to the North American Symptomatic Carotid Endarterectomy Trial (NASCET)[19], and these patients clearly benefit form carotid endarterectomy [19, 20]. Carotid stenting may be considered if surgery is deemed high risk [21, 22].

Spectral waveform assessment of the middle cerebral artery flow velocities (Figure 1.6)[23], emboli detection (Figure 1.7)[24], and vasomotor reactivity assessment (to be shown in subsequent chapters)[25, 26] with TCD can help identify patients who could be at higher risk of stroke recurrence. This information is complimentary to risk stratification or selection for revascularization based on the degree of the stenosis. I deploy these ultrasound tests to understand why TIA or stroke occurred, particularly if a patient was already receiving medical therapy currently deemed best for stroke prevention.

Another mechanism to consider across many patients, and particularly if the event occurred while on an antiplatelet agent, is cardiogenic embolism with conditions like atrial fibrillation that could be paroxysmal. Telemetry during the hospital stay and prolonged Holter-type (event detector) monitoring after discharge are helpful tools to detect atrial fibrillation. Electrocardiogram, if abnormal in our patient, should lend further support to pursue perhaps not only transthoracic (TTE) but also transesophageal echocardiography (TEE). Sonographers should be aware of possible paroxysmal dysrhythmias and should document an abnormal heart rhythm (Figure 1.8) apart from extra-systoli when seen during ultrasound tests – this would further raise suspicion for a cardioembolic mechanism of the event.

Lacunar, or small-vessel mechanism, should be considered next if DWI shows an appropriate small lesion in subcortical areas of white matter tracks and basal ganglia (Figure 1.9). However, despite such a convincing finding, other mechanisms should be considered because a small embolus can produce a subcortical or posterior circulation lesion mimicking lacune. Prognosis of a truly lacunar event is good but it should not preclude the workup for other risk factors that could be modifiable and that may necessitate treatment with more than aspirin and a statin.

Finally, less-common causes, such as an arterial dissection, paradoxical embolism, hypercoagulable state, etc., should be considered if the initial workup is negative for the more common mechanisms. Clues like recent trauma to the head and neck, events shortly after periods of prolonged immobility or trauma to the legs, unexplained weight loss, or

(*Continued*)

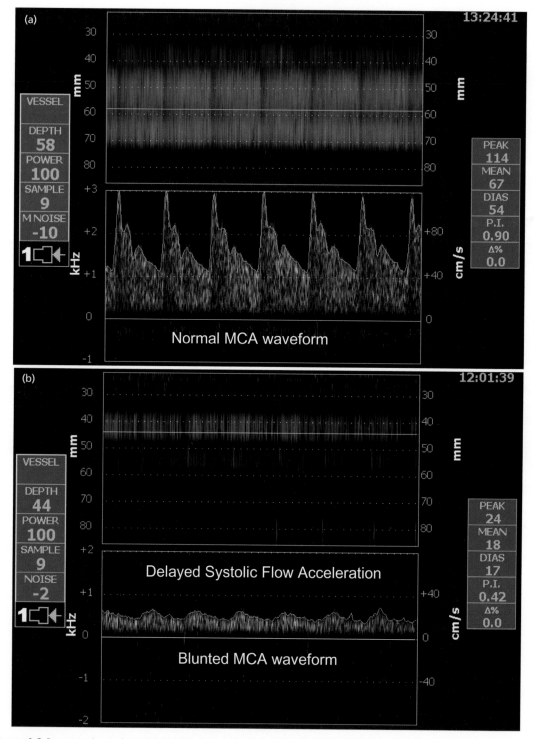

Figure 1.6 Power motion and spectral Doppler appearance of the normal and blunted MCA waveforms on transcranial Doppler. The upper part of (**a**) represents normal MCA appearance on motion display (vertical axis is the depth of insonation from the temporal window on the skull in mm). The lower part of (**a**) shows a typical spectral Doppler waveforms in the MCA with normal proximal ICA patency. (**b**) MCA appearance on motion display and spectral Doppler waveforms with hemodynamically significant ICA obstruction.

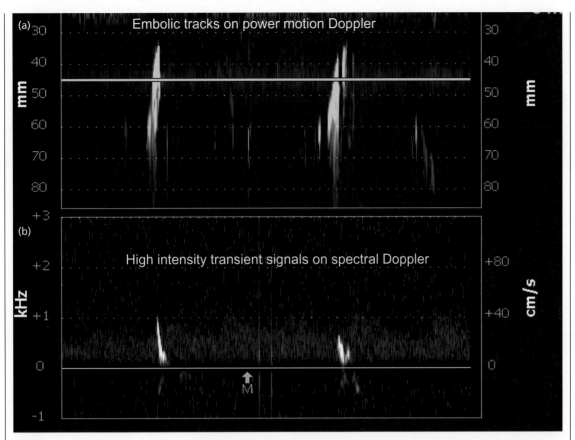

Figure 1.7 Embolic signals on power motion Doppler TCD. (**a**) The power motion display tracks emboli as they travel along cerebral vessels in real time (note the incline of tracks from right to left because the horizontal axis represents time and vertical axis represents the depth of vessel location in mm). (**b**) A spectral Doppler display of emboli at a single depth of insonation (the yellow line across motion display above).

recent history of deep venous thrombosis point to the need to consider such mechanisms. Additional vascular imaging, such as fat-suppression T2 MRI sequence, CTA, catheter angiography, and TCD emboli detection testing with agitated saline [27] (used as an echocontrast that is filtered out by lungs but detectable in the intracranial vessels in the presence of a right-to-left shunt), are helpful in these situations.

Upon completion of the diagnostic workup of our Case 1.1, a severe internal carotid artery (ICA) stenosis was found on carotid duplex corresponding to the 70–99% NASCET diameter reduction stenosis

range caused by a heterogeneous plaque with an irregular surface (Figure 1.4). His low-density lipoprotein (LDL) was 182; MRI DWI was negative. This patient had a TIA due to large-vessel atheromatous disease. He was given 325 mg aspirin and 80 mg atorvastatin in the emergency room. During TCD testing, one microembolic signal was seen after receiving aspirin. His case was discussed with the endovascular neurosurgeon and he also received 300 mg clopidogrel load while his carotid revascularization procedure was planned. The decision to add clopidogrel to aspirin prior to revascularization was based on the clinical trial evidence that dual antiplatelet therapy

(Continued)

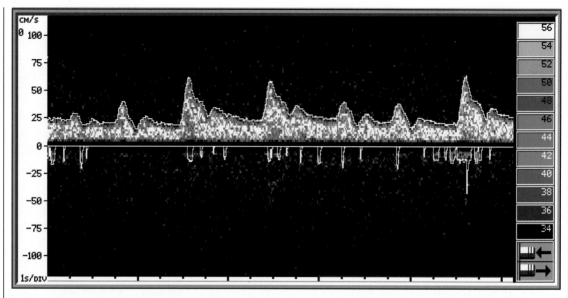

Figure 1.8 Atrial fibrillation appearance on spectral Doppler recording. Irregular-irregular rhythm recording was obtained from the MCA in a patient with acute stroke and paroxysmal atrial fibrillation. Sonographers should store abnormal waveforms like this if seen during diagnostic TCD or carotid duplex tests.

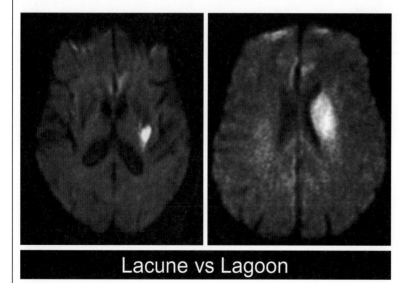

Figure 1.9 Typical lacunar stroke versus a subcortical infarction due to an embolus in the MCA.

reduce artery-to-artery embolization [28, 29], and differences in medical management in the CREST trial between surgical and stenting groups that could have led to higher perioperative myocardial ischemia events after carotid endarterectomy (CEA) on aspirin alone [22]. Carotid endarterectomy was done the next day. After surgery, he continued on clopidogrel and atorvastatin and he was encouraged to quit smoking. Of note, his ankle–brachial index (ABI) was 0.8.

Case study 1.2

A 70-year-old woman with a past medical history of arterial hypertension and coronary artery disease suddenly developed left-sided weakness. She called her daughter who then called 9-1-1 and the patient arrived 2 hours after symptom onset. Upon arrival, she reports that her strength has significantly improved mainly in her left hand. Her total NIHSS score is 2, for mild drift in the left arm and mild inattention to the left side with no gaze preference. Her symptoms continued to improve after CT scan, leaving her with only the drift at 2 hours and 25 minutes from symptom onset. No tissue plasminogen activator was given due to neurological improvement to a nondisabling level of the remaining symptoms. The patient passed the swallow test at bedside and was given 325 mg aspirin. She was then placed with the head of the bed flat and given 500 mL bolus of i.v. fluids. The patient was admitted to the Stroke Unit with neurological checks every hour for the next 6 hours, and every 2 hours thereafter for 24 hours. Her MRI at 4.5 hours from symptom onset showed a small cortical lesion on the DWI (Figure 1.10) that was also dark on the ADC sequence.

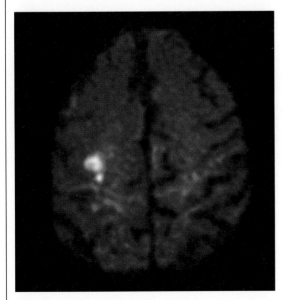

Figure 1.10 Small cortical lesion on DWI.

1. What is the diagnosis?
An acute ischemic stroke.

2. Should this patient have been offered reperfusion therapy?
Yes, if the remaining deficit after CT scan would still have been disabling, because the completeness of the "rapid" resolution of symptoms as a contraindication for intravenous tPA has not been defined or quantified.

3. What is the likely mechanism?
Likely an embolic event, either artery-to-artery or cardioembolic.

4. What is (are) the next test(s) that have the highest yield to identify this mechanism?
Carotid duplex to rule out carotid stenosis, and telemetry (admission ECG did not show atrial fibrillation (AFib)).

5. What are the risks for the patient now?
Neurological deterioration following spontaneous improvement or stroke progression/ recurrence.

6. What is the likelihood of such deterioration?
This clinical phenomenon has been reported in various trials and studies affecting as many as 13 to 37.5% of hyperacute stroke patients presenting within the time window for thrombolysis [30, 31].

7. What are the main predictors of possible deterioration following spontaneous improvement?
Persistence of an arterial occlusion, cardiac decompensation, early ischemic changes on admission CT scan, re-embolization/ re-occlusion, extension of an ischemic territory (stroke in evolution, brain swelling), baseline stroke severity, and elevated serum glucose [32–36].

8. What are the tests and their findings that can identify a patient at risk of stroke progression, recurrence or deterioration?
  • MRA, CTA, or catheter-angiography or TCD/ carotid duplex for the presence/ persistence of an occlusion/ high-grade stenosis at the level supplying more brain tissue as compared to the extent of the DWI lesion (remember there may be a mismatch between mild symptoms and a larger area at risk);

(Continued)

- perfusion deficit on MR greater than the DWI lesion;
- poor cardiac ejection fraction on echocardiography;
- arterial hypotension;
- embolic signals on TCD;
- diminished or exhausted vasomotor reactivity or intracranial arterial blood flow steal on TCD;
- the presence of a thrombus (with or without underlying atheromatous lesion) on carotid duplex or angiography.

The subsequent course and workup of our patient was as follows. Telemetry showed paroxysmal AFib, and repeated neurological examinations showed stable and complete symptom resolution. TCD at 8 hours from symptom onset showed complete spontaneous recanalization of the right M1 and proximal M2 middle cerebral artery (MCA) segments and no microembolic signals. Bed rest and flat head positioning were discontinued the next day. TEE showed a normal ejection fraction and no intracardiac thrombus. No heparin was administered. The patient was offered a direct thrombin inhibitor or warfarin for secondary stroke prevention in the setting of paroxysmal AFib and a small cortical stroke and no evidence of hemorrhagic transformation.

Case study 1.3

A 55-year-old man with a past medical history of diabetes and arterial hypertension noticed right-sided weakness when he woke up at night but chose not to call for help until the morning when he woke up completely flaccid on the right side. He was last seen normal at midnight the previous night, that is 7 hours before arrival to the hospital. Admission CT scan was normal with the Alberta Stroke Program Emergent CTScore (ASPECTS) of 10 points (Figure 1.11)[37]. (Figure 1.12, in contrast, shows an ASPECTS score of 1 where most areas of the middle cerebral artery territory are affected by early ischemic changes.) The NIHSS score was 8 points (pure motor weakness, arm equal to leg). No speech problems or other cortical signs were found.

1. What is the diagnosis?

Likely an acute ischemic stroke.

2. Why likely?

Since there is no intracranial bleeding and no hypoattenuation on head CT (given the time elapsed from last seen normal) to explain the patient's symptoms, there is a chance that it could be a stroke mimic.

3. If attributable to cerebral ischemia, what is the likely mechanism of this event?

Small-vessel or lacunar mechanism is likely in the setting of typical risk factors such as arterial hyper-tension and diabetes; however, other mechanisms should not be discounted.

4. What is (are) the test(s) that could help ascertain this mechanism or suspect others?

Since the patient presents 7 hours from last seen normal with definitely disabling deficit, emergent CTA of the head and neck or TCD and carotid duplex could be done to rule out an embolus or athero-thrombotic lesion potentially amenable to intervention (normal head CT within the time window for a thrombectomy device deployment) even though the clinical examination points to a subcortical lesion. A partially occlusive thrombus in the M1 MCA may initially cause hypoperfusion in the perforator(s) originating from the M1 segment. If vessels are patent, the next test should be MRI, because it would be the most sensitive test to confirm lacunar stroke in the acute setting.

5. If MRI shows a subcortical lesion, should the patient receive the rest of a standard workup including echocardiography, telemetry, etc.?

Yes, the standard workup should be completed because a small embolus can produce a subcortical lesion that could be confused with a lacune. A sub-cortical lesion affecting several perforating vessels is colloquially called a "lagoon" or "macune" (an example was shown in Figure 1.9, right image), and

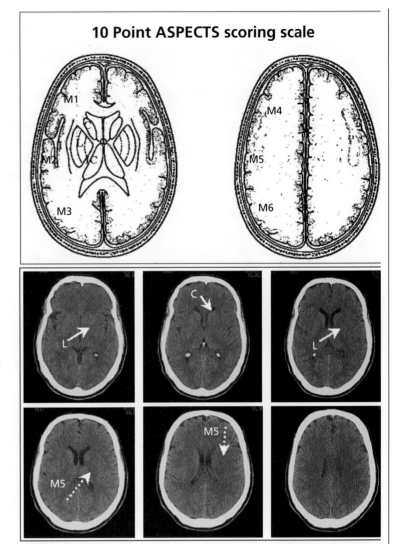

Figure 1.11 Alberta Stroke Program Emergent Computed Tomography Score (ASPECTS). A ten-point scoring system that focuses on the MCA territory over three ganglionic and three supraganglionic cuts. Each specific area is marked: I, insular ribbon; C, caudate nucleus; L, lentiform nucleus; IC, internal capsule; and M1, M2, M3, M4, M5, and M6 areas (this should not be confused with the order of MCA branches on angiography). If none are affected, the ASPECTS score is a maximum of 10 points.

this imaging finding should raise even more suspicion for possible embolic sources.

6. What if the DWI turns out to be negative?

If the DWI is negative and the patient's symptoms persist, it could be that time is needed for a small-vessel lesion to mature and appear on DWI [38] (sometimes it takes up to 3 days for a small lesion to appear on DWI particularly in the posterior circulation), or you may be dealing with hypoperfusion in the subcortical or posterior circulation area, or the patient has psychogenic symptoms.

The workup was completed and DWI showed a typical lacunar lesion while TCD in the emergency room was normal and so was the subsequent MRA. The patient was not currently taking aspirin, and he was given 325 mg on admission. He was then switched to aspirin plus extended-release dipyridamole for secondary stroke prevention. Tighter glycemic control and blood pressure medicines adjustment were recommended. He also was started on a statin.

(Continued)

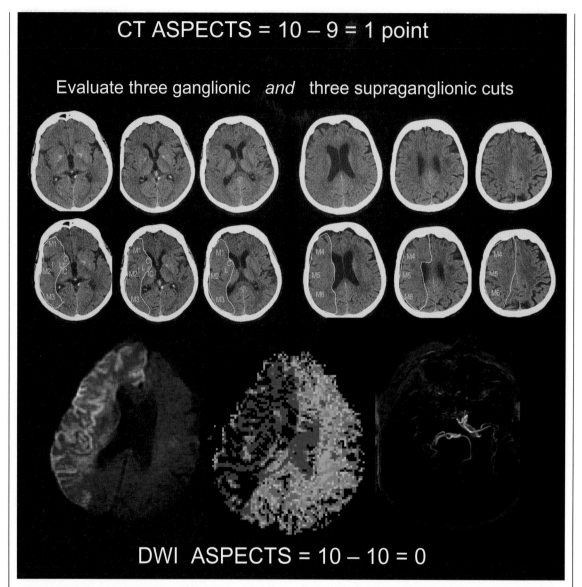

Figure 1.12 CT and MRI appearance of an extensive hemispheric ischemic lesion. All CT ASPECTS areas are affected by early ischemic changes except the internal capsule (images and interpretation courtesy of Andrew Demchuk, MD). For more information see www.aspectsinstroke.com (accessed Dec 11 2012). The bottom row of images show DWI, MR-perfusion, and MR-angiography findings in the patient with baseline ASPECTS score of 1.I, insular ribbon; C, caudate nucleus; L, lentiform nucleus; IC, internal capsule.

Case study 1.4

A 16-year-old female, who was taking a birth control pill and actively smoking, suddenly developed left-sided weakness (for additional discussion, see [39]). She was brought to an outside hospital and her CT scan was negative. The Emergency Medicine physician reported a focal neurological deficit with the total NIHSS score of 10 points at 2.5 hours from symptom onset. Even though the NINDS rt-PA Stroke Study did not enroll patients younger than 18 years of age, the disabling nature of the deficit in an adolescent prompted the decision to give intravenous tPA 0.9 mg/kg (10% bolus, 90% continuous infusion for 1 hour), and transfer her (or "drip'n ship") to the comprehensive stroke center. Upon arrival, and with tPA infusion just about to be completed, she regained most of her strength in the left side and still showed no cortical deficits (total NIHSS score of 4 points).

1. What is the diagnosis?

Despite her young age, it is likely an ischemic stroke due to her risk factors.

2. Should she be considered for additional catheter reperfusion?

Although the Interventional Management of Stroke (IMS) 3 trial [40] was stopped for futility, it did not properly test the latest technologies such as stentrievers [41]. Given her young age and the possibility of neurological worsening if the occlusion persists or the vessel re-occludes, an intra-arterial intervention (mechanical thrombus removal, i.e. thrombectomy) should be considered as an option. Urgent CTA of the head and neck or TCD will help determine if the MCA occlusion is still present. Rapid improvement during tPA infusion to the nondisabling level of her symptoms would be an argument against the risks

of an endovascular intervention. The management will change should neurological worsening occur due to re-occlusion.

3. What is likely the mechanism?

Differential for stroke in the young is long and among other conditions pertinent to our acute case it includes paradoxical embolism, dissection, cardiogenic embolism, hypercoagulable state, and moya-moya.

4. What is (are) the next test(s) to confirm ischemic etiology and determine the pathogenic mechanism? MRI of the brain and TCD "bubble" test (or emboli detection with intravenous contrast injection of 9 cc normal saline agitated with 1 cc room air)[27].

Her workup showed no ischemic changes on the noncontrast head CT upon arrival and patent right MCA at the end of the tPA infusion on TCD examination at bedside (Figure 1.13). Her TCD "bubble" test (or TCD emboli detection with contrast injection also done at the same time at the bedside, Figure 1.13) was positive for Spencer's grade III shunt at rest augmented to grade IV with Valsalva [42]. Her DWI showed a large subcortical ischemic lesion (or "lagoon"; Figure 1.14), and her MRA was normal. Her MRI sequences were extended to include a pelvic MR venogram that showed a thrombus (Figure 1.14). TEE showed patent foramen ovale (PFO)(Figure 1.14). She was instructed to quit smoking and stop taking the birth control pill. The risks and lack of evidence for PFO closure were discussed and she opted for closure of the shunt. She was started on 325 mg aspirin and 75 mg clopidogrel and received percutaneous PFO closure 1 month after her stroke. Her NIHSS was 0 and mRS was 0, and she gave birth to a healthy child 1 year later.

(Continued)

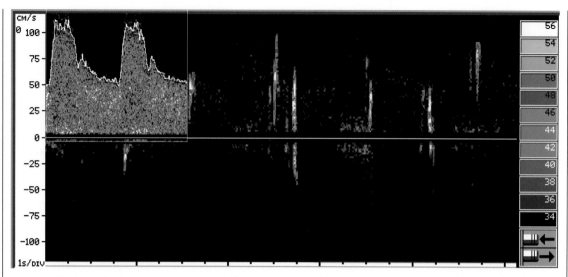

Figure 1.13 Spectral MCA waveform and embolic signals during TCD bubble test for right-to-left shunt. MCA waveforms (insert) are reflective of normal vessel patency. Air microbubble traces on spectral Doppler are seen as high-intensity transient signals (HITS). These HITS appeared after intravenous injection of agitated saline at rest. Gain was reduced to subtracted normal flow signals.

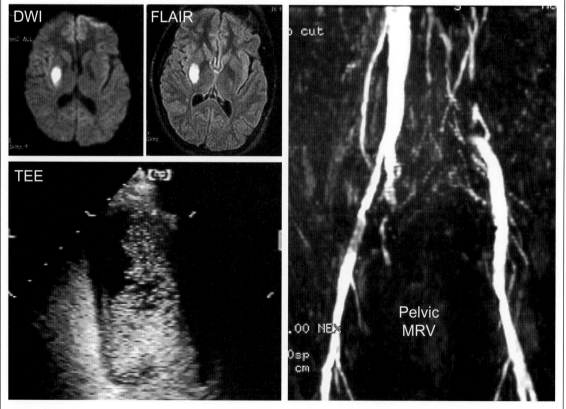

Figure 1.14 MRI findings in a young patient with paradoxical embolism and patent foramen ovale on transesophageal echocardiography (TEE). DWI and fluid-attenuated inversion recovery (FLAIR) show a subacute lesion despite complete symptom resolution at the time of MRI. MR venogram of the pelvis (right) shows flow void due to thrombus. TEE shows air bubble passage into the left ventricle after intravenous injection of agitated saline.

Case study 1.5

A 67-year-old man with a past medical history of coronary artery bypass graft (CABG), peripheral arterial disease, smoking (quit 3 years ago), and daytime sleepiness developed right-sided weakness 2 days ago that was getting worse at night/ morning and better during the day and that he attributed to his arthritis. He decided to seek help when his wife noticed the facial droop on the right and occasional problems finding the correct words. His NIHSS score was 3 upon arrival and his head CT showed a small cortical hypoattenuation in the left frontal lobe with no hemorrhage.

1. What is the diagnosis?

Subacute (greater than 24 hours from onset) ischemic stroke with fluctuating course and worsening of symptoms.

2. What is the likely mechanism?

This patient has polyvascular atheromatous disease, and carotid or intracranial stenoses should be suspected first. Although the course of his symptoms is not typical for an embolic stroke (when the symptoms are often most severe at onset followed by improvement as the embolus dissolves and moves distally), cardioembolism should still be a suspect. Finally, the presence of cortical symptoms (mild aphasia) argues against the small-vessel mechanism.

3. Which is (are) the test(s) that can help determine pathogenic mechanism?

MRI, carotid duplex, TCD, and CTA (if MRA/ultrasound results are discrepant) as well as telemetry and echocardiography should all be done because you suspect either hemodynamic changes in the setting or an extra- or intracranial stenosis, or artery-to-artery embolism, or cardiac embolism. Fluctuating symptoms are likely attributable to changing perfusion pressures and collateral supply rather then recurrent embolization into the same arterial territory. If telemetry is negative, this patient should also be referred for 1-month event detection (prolonged Holter monitoring) to detect paroxysmal atrial fibrillation.

4. Because the patient's symptoms fluctuate and worsen, should reperfusion therapy be considered?

This patient presents outside conventional time windows for systemic thrombolysis and towards the end of timeframes currently considered for endovascular interventions, that is 8 hours from symptom onset. At the moment, he has relatively mild deficit (right arm drift, mild word-finding difficulty and right facial droop). Consider the underlying mechanism of neurological fluctuation, such as a high-grade stenosis or an embolus. If found, these would indicate the possibility of clinical worsening to the point of a clearly debilitating deficit, which would justify the risk of endovascular reperfusion. The probability of neurological worsening can also be demonstrated by a perfusion defect on MRI or CT-perfusion larger than the hypoattenuation area on CT or a lesion on DWI. In parallel with consideration of aggressive reperfusion strategies and further multimodal imaging of a patient with mild deficits, medical management should be optimized, that is place with the head of the bed flat or even Tredelen-burg, hydration with intravenous fluids, clopidogrel 300 mg load (he has been taking 81 mg of aspirin only), atorvastatin 80 mg, glycemic control, etc. On admission, his blood pressure should not be lowered (unless it exceeds 220/120 mmHg) until vascular imaging is completed and the mechanism of fluctuation/worsening is ascertained. I use bedside carotid duplex and TCD as an extension of my neurological examination to obtain the pathophysiological information in real time. Multimodal MRI/MRA or CTA/ CTP can provide insights into the pathogenesis of his symptoms but lack information about vasomotor reactivity, recruitment of collaterals, and continuing embolization – information easily derived from the ultrasound tests.

5. What if both a significant carotid stenosis and atrial fibrillation are found in this patient?

If carotid duplex or angiography show ≥50% left ICA stenosis and telemetry reveals paroxysmal atrial fibrillation, both of these conditions can produce ischemic stroke and it would be hard to decide which one is the leading cause. If both conditions, each of which could lead to stroke, are confirmed, the patient's pathogenic mechanism of stroke is still deemed to be undetermined [12]. Secondary prevention strategies should nonetheless account for

(Continued)

both, that is this patient may be considered for carotid revascularization and take both an anticoagulant and an antiplatelet agent long term.

Upon completion of the diagnostic workup, a severe (70–99% NASCET range) stenosis was found on carotid duplex by the multidisciplinary consensus criteria [43] and telemetry showed paroxysmal atrial fibrillation. Applying TOAST the classification [12], the pathogenic mechanism remains cryptogenic or undetermined. However, the workup revealed risk factors that can be addressed. First, the patient is a candidate for carotid endarterectomy (CEA) or stenting (CAS) because he has a severe symptomatic carotid stenosis. Second, carotid revascularization should be done within 2 weeks of the stroke symptom onset to maximize the protective effect of carotid revascularization, as shown in CEA trials [44]. After carotid revascularization, the patient should receive anticoagulation (a direct thrombin inhibitor or war-

farin) because paroxysmal atrial fibrillation places him at practically the same risk of ischemic stroke as persistent or permanent atrial fibrillation [45]. He also should continue on clopidogrel (without aspirin or with aspirin if stenting was performed) due to peripheral arterial disease and coronary artery disease. Unlike preventative measures after acute coronary syndrome, ischemic stroke patients are at a higher risk of bleeding on dual antiplatelet therapy long term in the absence of a larger stroke prevention benefit [46]. Short-term use of dual antiplatelet therapy may be advisable before CEA. Furthermore, blood pressure and lipid-lowering therapies as well as strict glycemic control, should be continued. The patient should receive a referral for a sleep study because sleep apnea is common among patients with stroke and can increase the risk of stroke, myocardial infarction, and sudden death, and it makes BP and glucose management more difficult [47].

These cases represent some of the many considerations that vascular neurologists have when we evaluate and manage patients with stroke and TIA. Imagine now how the pace of the evaluation and workup changes when patients arrive acutely, and quick decisions have to be made on how to reverse the stroke or stop worsening/ fluctuation with much less information at hand and with tools that have to be available in an emergency. The next chapter addresses how time becomes important for the brain to survive when ischemia starts because tissues become at risk of completing infarction and chaos increases when entropy follows the arrow of time. Meanwhile, time is also relative as every patient enters ischemia with different risk factors, abilities to collateralize, as well as differences is size and composition of the thromboembolic material and the location of steno-occlusive lesions. Real-time pathophysiological assessment provides clues as to what is happening and how each individual patient has a unique set of circumstances that may help tailor our management decisions.

Appendix 1.1 The National Institutes of Health Stroke Scale (NIHSS) score

(source: www.ninds.nih.gov/doctors/NIH_Stroke_Scale.pdf; accessed Dec 11, 2012).

Note: the NIHSS is not a substitute for a complete neurological examination. NIHSS is used in emergency situations to document the severity of an ischemic stroke by assessing typical functions most commonly affected by the stroke. If NIHSS is 0 but the patient has neurological deficits, it is likely due to the fact that not all deficits are included into the NIHSS. For example, isolated diplopia, agraphia, acalculia, or thalamic pain. If a deficit cannot be scored, your assessment should document if this neurological problem is present and if it is disabling or not. The presence of a disabling deficit should prompt consideration of reperfusion therapies.

Furthermore, the NIHSS score was not developed for assessment and prognostication of the intracerebral hemorrhage (ICH). Though also applied to patients with ICH to document the severity of the neurological deficit, it should not be used in isolation. The well-established predictors of outcomes after ICH should be documented such as the Glasgow Coma Scale (GCS), ICH volume (cc), location (supra- or infratentorial, deep or lobar), and the presence of an intraventricular extension.

N I H
STROKE
SCALE

Patient Identification. ___ ___-___ ___ ___-___ ___ ___

Pt. Date of Birth ___ ___/___ ___/___ ___

Hospital _____(___ ___-___ ___)

Date of Exam ___ ___/___ ___/___ ___

Interval: [ ] Baseline   [ ] 2 hours post treatment   [ ] 24 hours post onset of symptoms ±20 minutes   [ ] 7-10 days
      [ ] 3 months   [ ] Other _____(___ ___)

Time: ___ ___:___ ___   [ ]am [ ]pm

Person Administering Scale _____

Administer stroke scale items in the order listed. Record performance in each category after each subscale exam. Do not go back and change scores. Follow directions provided for each exam technique. Scores should reflect what the patient does, not what the clinician thinks the patient can do. The clinician should record answers while administering the exam and work quickly. Except where indicated, the patient should not be coached (i.e., repeated requests to patient to make a special effort).

Instructions	Scale Definition	Score
1a. Level of Consciousness: The investigator must choose a response if a full evaluation is prevented by such obstacles as an endotracheal tube, language barrier, orotracheal trauma/bandages. A 3 is scored only if the patient makes no movement (other than reflexive posturing) in response to noxious stimulation.	0 = **Alert;** keenly responsive. 1 = **Not alert**; but arousable by minor stimulation to obey, answer, or respond. 2 = **Not alert**; requires repeated stimulation to attend, or is obtunded and requires strong or painful stimulation to make movements (not stereotyped). 3 = Responds only with reflex motor or autonomic effects or totally unresponsive, flaccid, and areflexic.	_____
1b. LOC Questions: The patient is asked the month and his/her age. The answer must be correct - there is no partial credit for being close. Aphasic and stuporous patients who do not comprehend the questions will score 2. Patients unable to speak because of endotracheal intubation, orotracheal trauma, severe dysarthria from any cause, language barrier, or any other problem not secondary to aphasia are given a 1. It is important that only the initial answer be graded and that the examiner not "help" the patient with verbal or non-verbal cues.	0 = **Answers** both questions correctly. 1 = **Answers** one question correctly. 2 = **Answers** neither question correctly.	_____
1c. LOC Commands: The patient is asked to open and close the eyes and then to grip and release the non-paretic hand. Substitute another one step command if the hands cannot be used. Credit is given if an unequivocal attempt is made but not completed due to weakness. If the patient does not respond to command, the task should be demonstrated to him or her (pantomime), and the result scored (i.e., follows none, one or two commands). Patients with trauma, amputation, or other physical impediments should be given suitable one-step commands. Only the first attempt is scored.	0 = **Performs** both tasks correctly. 1 = **Performs** one task correctly. 2 = **Performs** neither task correctly.	_____
2. Best Gaze: Only horizontal eye movements will be tested. Voluntary or reflexive (oculocephalic) eye movements will be scored, but caloric testing is not done. If the patient has a conjugate deviation of the eyes that can be overcome by voluntary or reflexive activity, the score will be 1. If a patient has an isolated peripheral nerve paresis (CN III, IV or VI), score a 1. Gaze is testable in all aphasic patients. Patients with ocular trauma, bandages, pre-existing blindness, or other disorder of visual acuity or fields should be tested with reflexive movements, and a choice made by the investigator. Establishing eye contact and then moving about the patient from side to side will occasionally clarify the presence of a partial gaze palsy.	0 = **Normal.** 1 = **Partial gaze palsy;** gaze is abnormal in one or both eyes, but forced deviation or total gaze paresis is not present. 2 = **Forced deviation,** or total gaze paresis not overcome by the oculocephalic maneuver.	_____

N I H
STROKE
SCALE

Patient Identification. ___ __-__ __ __-__ __ __

Pt. Date of Birth ___ __/__ __/__ __

Hospital _____ (__ __-__ __)

Date of Exam ___ __/__ __/__ __

Interval: [ ] Baseline [ ] 2 hours post treatment [ ] 24 hours post onset of symptoms ±20 minutes [ ] 7-10 days
[ ] 3 months [ ] Other _____(__ __)

3. Visual: Visual fields (upper and lower quadrants) are tested by confrontation, using finger counting or visual threat, as appropriate. Patients may be encouraged, but if they look at the side of the moving fingers appropriately, this can be scored as normal. If there is unilateral blindness or enucleation, visual fields in the remaining eye are scored. Score 1 only if a clear-cut asymmetry, including quadrantanopia, is found. If patient is blind from any cause, score 3. Double simultaneous stimulation is performed at this point. If there is extinction, patient receives a 1, and the results are used to respond to item 11.	0 = **No visual loss.** 1 = **Partial hemianopia.** 2 = **Complete hemianopia.** 3 = **Bilateral hemianopia** (blind including cortical blindness).	____
4. Facial Palsy: Ask – or use pantomime to encourage – the patient to show teeth or raise eyebrows and close eyes. Score symmetry of grimace in response to noxious stimuli in the poorly responsive or non-comprehending patient. If facial trauma/bandages, orotracheal tube, tape or other physical barriers obscure the face, these should be removed to the extent possible.	0 = **Normal** symmetrical movements. 1 = **Minor paralysis** (flattened nasolabial fold, asymmetry on smiling). 2 = **Partial paralysis** (total or near-total paralysis of lower face). 3 = **Complete paralysis** of one or both sides (absence of facial movement in the upper and lower face).	____
5. Motor Arm: The limb is placed in the appropriate position: extend the arms (palms down) 90 degrees (if sitting) or 45 degrees (if supine). Drift is scored if the arm falls before 10 seconds. The aphasic patient is encouraged using urgency in the voice and pantomime, but not noxious stimulation. Each limb is tested in turn, beginning with the non-paretic arm. Only in the case of amputation or joint fusion at the shoulder, the examiner should record the score as untestable (UN), and clearly write the explanation for this choice.	0 = **No drift;** limb holds 90 (or 45) degrees for full 10 seconds. 1 = **Drift;** limb holds 90 (or 45) degrees, but drifts down before full 10 seconds; does not hit bed or other support. 2 = **Some effort against gravity;** limb cannot get to or maintain (if cued) 90 (or 45) degrees, drifts down to bed, but has some effort against gravity. 3 = **No effort against gravity;** limb falls. 4 = **No movement.** UN = **Amputation** or joint fusion, explain: _____ **5a. Left Arm** **5b. Right Arm**	 ____ ____
6. Motor Leg: The limb is placed in the appropriate position: hold the leg at 30 degrees (always tested supine). Drift is scored if the leg falls before 5 seconds. The aphasic patient is encouraged using urgency in the voice and pantomime, but not noxious stimulation. Each limb is tested in turn, beginning with the non-paretic leg. Only in the case of amputation or joint fusion at the hip, the examiner should record the score as untestable (UN), and clearly write the explanation for this choice.	0 = **No drift;** leg holds 30-degree position for full 5 seconds. 1 = **Drift;** leg falls by the end of the 5-second period but does not hit bed. 2 = **Some effort against gravity;** leg falls to bed by 5 seconds, but has some effort against gravity. 3 = **No effort against gravity;** leg falls to bed immediately. 4 = **No movement.** UN = **Amputation** or joint fusion, explain: _____ **6a. Left Leg** **6b. Right Leg**	 ____

N I H STROKE SCALE

Patient Identification. ___ ___-___ ___-___ ___

Pt. Date of Birth ___ __/___ __/___ ___

Hospital _____(__ __-__ __)

Date of Exam ___ __/___ __/___ ___

Interval: [ ] Baseline   [ ] 2 hours post treatment   [ ] 24 hours post onset of symptoms ±20 minutes   [ ] 7-10 days
[ ] 3 months   [ ] Other _____(__ __)

7. Limb Ataxia: This item is aimed at finding evidence of a unilateral cerebellar lesion. Test with eyes open. In case of visual defect, ensure testing is done in intact visual field. The finger-nose-finger and heel-shin tests are performed on both sides, and ataxia is scored only if present out of proportion to weakness. Ataxia is absent in the patient who cannot understand or is paralyzed. Only in the case of amputation or joint fusion, the examiner should record the score as untestable (UN), and clearly write the explanation for this choice. In case of blindness, test by having the patient touch nose from extended arm position.	0 = **Absent.** 1 = **Present in one limb.** 2 = **Present in two limbs.** UN = **Amputation** or joint fusion, explain: _____	_____
8. Sensory: Sensation or grimace to pinprick when tested, or withdrawal from noxious stimulus in the obtunded or aphasic patient. Only sensory loss attributed to stroke is scored as abnormal and the examiner should test as many body areas (arms [not hands], legs, trunk, face) as needed to accurately check for hemisensory loss. A score of 2, "severe or total sensory loss," should only be given when a severe or total loss of sensation can be clearly demonstrated. Stuporous and aphasic patients will, therefore, probably score 1 or 0. The patient with brainstem stroke who has bilateral loss of sensation is scored 2. If the patient does not respond and is quadriplegic, score 2. Patients in a coma (item 1a=3) are automatically given a 2 on this item.	0 = **Normal;** no sensory loss. 1 = **Mild-to-moderate sensory loss;** patient feels pinprick is less sharp or is dull on the affected side; or there is a loss of superficial pain with pinprick, but patient is aware of being touched. 2 = **Severe to total sensory loss;** patient is not aware of being touched in the face, arm, and leg.	_____
9. Best Language: A great deal of information about comprehension will be obtained during the preceding sections of the examination. For this scale item, the patient is asked to describe what is happening in the attached picture, to name the items on the attached naming sheet and to read from the attached list of sentences. Comprehension is judged from responses here, as well as to all of the commands in the preceding general neurological exam. If visual loss interferes with the tests, ask the patient to identify objects placed in the hand, repeat, and produce speech. The intubated patient should be asked to write. The patient in a coma (item 1a=3) will automatically score 3 on this item. The examiner must choose a score for the patient with stupor or limited cooperation, but a score of 3 should be used only if the patient is mute and follows no one-step commands.	0 = **No aphasia;** normal. 1 = **Mild-to-moderate aphasia;** some obvious loss of fluency or facility of comprehension, without significant limitation on ideas expressed or form of expression. Reduction of speech and/or comprehension, however, makes conversation about provided materials difficult or impossible. For example, in conversation about provided materials, examiner can identify picture or naming card content from patient's response. 2 = **Severe aphasia;** all communication is through fragmentary expression; great need for inference, questioning, and guessing by the listener. Range of information that can be exchanged is limited; listener carries burden of communication. Examiner cannot identify materials provided from patient response. 3 = **Mute, global aphasia;** no usable speech or auditory comprehension.	_____
10. Dysarthria: If patient is thought to be normal, an adequate sample of speech must be obtained by asking patient to read or repeat words from the attached list. If the patient has severe aphasia, the clarity of articulation of spontaneous speech can be rated. Only if the patient is intubated or has other physical barriers to producing speech, the examiner should record the score as untestable (UN), and clearly write an explanation for this choice. Do not tell the patient why he or she is being tested.	0 = **Normal.** 1 = **Mild-to-moderate dysarthria;** patient slurs at least some words and, at worst, can be understood with some difficulty. 2 = **Severe dysarthria;** patient's speech is so slurred as to be unintelligible in the absence of or out of proportion to any dysphasia, or is mute/anarthric. UN = **Intubated** or other physical barrier, explain:_____	_____

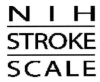

Patient Identification. ___ ___-___ ___ ___-___ ___ ___

Pt. Date of Birth ___ ___/___ ___/___ ___

Hospital _____(___ ___-___ ___)

Date of Exam ___ ___/___ ___/___ ___

Interval: [ ] Baseline   [ ] 2 hours post treatment   [ ] 24 hours post onset of symptoms ±20 minutes   [ ] 7-10 days
          [ ] 3 months   [ ] Other _____(___ ___)

| **11. Extinction and Inattention (formerly Neglect):** Sufficient information to identify neglect may be obtained during the prior testing. If the patient has a severe visual loss preventing visual double simultaneous stimulation, and the cutaneous stimuli are normal, the score is normal. If the patient has aphasia but does appear to attend to both sides, the score is normal. The presence of visual spatial neglect or anosagnosia may also be taken as evidence of abnormality. Since the abnormality is scored only if present, the item is never untestable. | 0 = **No abnormality.**

1 = **Visual, tactile, auditory, spatial, or personal inattention** or extinction to bilateral simultaneous stimulation in one of the sensory modalities.

2 = **Profound hemi-inattention or extinction to more than one modality;** does not recognize own hand or orients to only one side of space. | _____ |

_____
_____

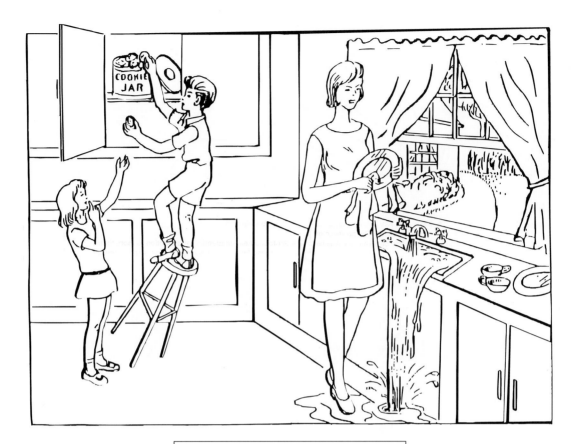

You know how.

Down to earth.

I got home from work.

Near the table in the dining room.

They heard him speak on the radio last night.

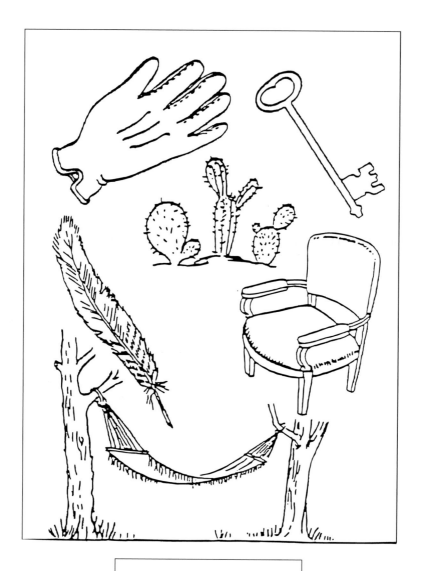

MAMA

TIP – TOP

FIFTY – FIFTY

THANKS

HUCKLEBERRY

BASEBALL PLAYER

References

1. Astrup J, Symon L, Branston NM, *et al.* Cortical evoked potential and extracellular K^+ and H^+ at critical levels of brain ischemia. *Stroke* 1977; **8**: 51–7.

2. Trojaborg W, Boysen G. Relation between EEG, regional cerebral blood flow and internal carotid stump pressure during carotid endarterectomy. *Electroencephalogr Clin Neurophysiol* 1973; **34**: 61–9.

3. Heiss WD, Waltz AG, Hayakawa T. Neuronal function and local blood flow during experimental cerebral ischemia. In: Harper AM, Jennett WB, Miller JD, *et al.* (eds), *Blood Flow and Metabolism in the Brain*. Edinburgh: Churchill Livingstone, 1975, pp. 14–27.

4. Branston NM, Symon L, Crockard HA, *et al.* Relationship between the cortical evoked potential and local cortical blood flow following acute middle cerebral artery occlusion in the baboon. *Exp Neurol* 1974; **45**: 195–208.

5. Astrup J, Siesjo BK, Symon L. Thresholds in cerebral ischemia – the ischemic penumbra. *Stroke* 1981; **12**: 723–5.

6. Jones TH, Morawetz RB, Crowell RM, *et al.* Thresholds of focal cerebral ischemia in awake monkeys. *J Neurosurg* 1981; **54**: 773–82.

7. Hossman KA. Viability thresholds and the penumbra of focal ischemia. *Ann Neurol* 2004; **36**: 557–65.

8. Liebeskind DS. Time is brain – revisited. In: Liebeskind DS (ed.), *Diagnostic Strategies in Cerebral Ischemia*. Oxford: Clinical Publishing, 2011, pp.13–22.

9. Hacke W, Donnan G, Fieschi C, *et al.* Association of outcome with early stroke treatment: pooled analysis of ATLANTIS, ECASS, and NINDS rt-PA stroke trials. *Lancet* 2004; **363**: 768–74.

10. Adams HP Jr, Bendixen BH, Kappelle LJ, *et al.* Classification of subtype of acute ischemic stroke. Definitions for use in a multicenter clinical trial. TOAST. Trial of Org 10172 in Acute Stroke Treatment. *Stroke* 1993; **24**: 35–41.

11. Albers GW, Thijs VN, Wechsler L, *et al.* Magnetic resonance imaging profiles predict clinical response to early reperfusion: the diffusion and perfusion imaging evaluation for understanding stroke evolution (DEFUSE) study. *Ann Neurol* 2006; **60**: 508–17.

12. Johnston SC, Rothwell PM, Nguyen-Huynh MN, *et al.* Validation and refinement of scores to predict very early stroke risk after transient ischemic attack. *Lancet* 2007; **369**: 283–92.

13. Easton JD, Saver JL, Albers GW, *et al.* American Heart Association; American Stroke Association Stroke Council; Council on Cardiovascular Surgery and Anesthesia; Council on Cardiovascular Radiology and Intervention; Council on Cardiovascular Nursing; Interdisciplinary Council on Peripheral Vascular Disease. Definition and evaluation of transient ischemic attack: a scientific statement for healthcare professionals from the American Heart Association/American Stroke Association Stroke Council; Council on Cardiovascular Surgery and Anesthesia; Council on Cardiovascular Radiology and Intervention; Council on Cardiovascular Nursing; and the Interdisciplinary Council on Peripheral Vascular Disease. The American Academy of Neurology affirms the value of this statement as an educational tool for neurologists. *Stroke* 2009; **40**: 2276–93.

14. Coutts SB, Eliasziw M, Hill MD, *et al.* An improved scoring system for identifying patients at high early risk of stroke and functional impairment after an acute transient ischemic attack or minor stroke. *Intl J Stroke* 2008; **3**: 3–10.

15. Coutts SB, Simon JE, Eliasziw M, *et al.* triaging transient ischemic attack and minor stroke using acute magnetic resonance imaging. *Ann Neurol* 2005; **57**: 848–54.

16. Mast H, Thompson JL, Lin IF, *et al.* Cigarette smoking as a determinant of high-grade carotid artery stenosis in Hispanic, black, and white patients with stroke or transient ischemic attack. *Stroke* 1998; **29**: 908–12.

17. Wong KS, Huang YN, Gao S, *et al.* Intracranial stenosis in Chinese patients with acute stroke. *Neurology* 1998; **50**: 812–3.

18. Waddy SP, Cotsonis G, Lynn MJ, *et al.* Racial differences in vascular risk factors and outcomes of patients with intracranial atherosclerotic arterial stenosis. *Stroke* 2009; **40**: 719–25.

19. NASCET Collaborators. Benefit of carotid endarterectomy in patients with synmptomatic moderate or severe stenosis. *N Engl J Med* 1998; **339**: 1415–25.

20. ECST Collaborative Group. Randomised trial of endarterectomy for recently symptomatic carotid stenosis: final results of the MRC European Carotid Surgery Trial. *Lancet* 1998; **351**: 1379–87.

21. Yadav JS, Wholey MH, Kuntz RE, *et al.* SAPPHIRE Investigators. Protected carotid-artery stenting versus endarterectomy in high-risk patients. *N Engl J Med* 2004; **351**: 1493–1501.

22. Brott TG, Hobson RW, Howard G, *et al.* Stenting versus endarterectomy for treatment of carotid-artery stenosis (CREST). *N Engl J Med* 2010; **363**: 11–23.

23. Alexandrov AV, Sloan MA, Tegeler CH, *et al.* for the American Society of Neuroimaging Practice Guidelines Committee. Practice standards for transcranial Doppler (TCD) ultrasound. Part II. Clinical indications and expected outcomes. *J Neuroimaging* 2012; **22**: 215–24.

24. King A, Markus HS. Doppler embolic signals in cerebrovascular disease and prediction of stroke risk: a systematic review and meta-analysis. *Stroke* 2009; **40**: 3711–17.

25. Markus HS, Harrison MJ. Estimation of cerebrovascular reactivity using transcranial Doppler, including the use of breath-holding as the vasodilatory stimulus. *Stroke* 1992; **23**: 668–73.

26. Silvestrini M, Vernieri F, Pasqualetti P, *et al*. Impaired vasosmotor reactivity and risk of stroke in patients with asymptomatic carotid artery stenosis. *JAMA* 2000; **283**: 2122–7.

27. Jauss M, Zanette E. Detection of right to left shunt with ultrasound contrast agent and transcranial Doppler sonography. *Cerebrovasc Dis* 2000; **10**: 490–6.

28. Markus HS, Droste DW, Kaps M, *et al*. Dual antiplatelet therapy with clopidogrel and aspirin in symptomatic carotid stenosis evaluated using doppler embolic signal detection: the Clopidogrel and Aspirin for Reduction of Emboli in Symptomatic Carotid Stenosis (CARESS) trial. *Circulation* 2005; **111**: 2233–40.

29. Wong KS, Chen C, Fu J, *et al*. for the CLAIR study investigators. Clopidogrel plus aspirin versus aspirin alone for reducing embolisation in patients with acute symptomatic cerebral or carotid artery tenosis (CLAIR study): a randomised, open-label, blinded-endpoint trial. *Lancet Neurol* 2010; **9**: 489–97.

30. Dávalos A, Toni D, Iweins F, *et al*. Neurological deterioration in acute ischemic stroke: potential predictors and associated factors in the European cooperative acute stroke study (ECASS) I. *Stroke* 1999; **30**: 2631–6.

31. Grotta JC, Welch KM, Fagan SC, *et al*. Clinical deterioration following improvement in the NINDS rt-PA Stroke Trial. *Stroke* 2001; **32**: 661–8.

32. Irino T, Watanabe M, Nishide M, *et al*. Angiographical analysis of acute cerebral infarction followed by "cascade"-like deterioration of minor neurological deficits. What is progressing stroke? *Stroke* 1983; **14**: 363–8.

33. Bladin CF, Chambers BR. Frequency and pathogenesis of hemodynamic stroke. *Stroke* 1994; **25**: 2179–82.

34. Toni D, Fiorelli M, Gentile M, *et al*. Progressing neurological deficit secondary to acute ischemic stroke. A study on predictability, pathogenesis, and prognosis. *Arch Neurol* 1995; **52**: 670–5.

35. Toni D, Fiorelli M, Zanette EM, *et al*. Early spontaneous improvement and deterioration of ischemic stroke patients. A serial study with transcranial Doppler ultrasonography. *Stroke* 1998; **29**: 1144–8.

36. Alexandrov AV, Felberg RA, Demchuk AM, *et al*. Deterioration following spontaneous improvement: sonographic findings in patients with acutely resolving symptoms of cerebral ischemia. *Stroke* 2000; **31**: 915–19.

37. Barber PA, Demchuk AM, Zhang J, *et al*. Validity and reliability of a quantitative computed tomography score in predicting outcome of hyperacute stroke before thrombolytic therapy. ASPECTS Study Group. Alberta Stroke Programme Early CT Score. *Lancet* 2000; **355**: 1670–4.

38. Sylaja PN, Coutts SB, Krol A, *et al*. VISION Study Group. When to expect negative diffusion-weighted images in stroke and transient ischemic attack. *Stroke* 2008; **39**: 1898–900.

39. Noser E, Felberg RA, Alexandrov AV. Thrombolytic therapy in an adolescent ischemic stroke. *J Child Neurol* 2001; **16**: 286–8.

40. Broderick JP, Palesch YY, Demchuk AM, *et al*. the Interventional Management of Stroke (IMS) III Investigators. Endovascular Therapy after Intravenous t-PA versus t-PA Alone for Stroke. *N Engl J Med* 2013;DOI: 10.1056/NEJMoa1214300

41. Saver JL, Jahan R, Levy EI, *et al*. for the SWIFT Trialists. Solitaire flow restoration device versus the Merci Retriever in patients with acute ischaemic stroke (SWIFT): a randomised, parallel-group, non-inferiority trial. *Lancet* 2012; **380**:1241–9.

42. Spencer MP, Moehring MA, Jesurum J, *et al*. Power M mode transcranial doppler for diagnosis of patent foramen ovale and assessing transcatheter closure. *J Neuroimaging* 2004; **14**: 342–9.

43. Grant EG, Benson CB, Moneta GL, *et al*. Carotid artery stenosis: gray-scale and Doppler US diagnosis. Society of Radiologists in Ultrasound Consensus Conference. *Radiology* 2003; **229**: 340–6.

44. Rothwell PM, Eliasziw M, Gutnikov SA, *et al*. Carotid Endarterectomy Trialists Collaboration. Endarterectomy for symptomatic carotid stenosis in relation to clinical subgroups and timing of surgery. *Lancet* 2004; **363**: 915–24.

45. Chiang CE, Naditch-Brûlé L, Murin J, *et al*. Distribution and risk profile of paroxysmal, persistent, and permanent atrial fibrillation in routine clinical practice: insight from the real-life global survey evaluating patients with atrial fibrillation international registry. *Circ Arrhythm Electrophysiol* 2012; **5**: 632–9.

46. Bhatt DL, Fox KA, Hacke W, *et al*. CHARISMA Investigators. Clopidogrel and aspirin versus aspirin alone for the prevention of atherothrombotic events. *N Engl J Med* 2006; **354**: 1706–17.

47. Yaggi HK, Concato J, Kernan WN, *et al*. Obstructive sleep apnea as a risk factor for stroke and death. *N Engl J Med* 2005; **353**: 2034–41.

2 Time Is Brain and Brain Is Flow!

"I wasted time, and now doth time waste me."
William Shakespeare, *Richard II*

Our bodies change along the arrow of time from past to future, and when brain tissues become ischemic there is no time to waste, neither by stroke victims nor clinicians. The "Time is Brain!" mantra emerged from observations of the natural history of stroke and the overall time-sensitive efficacy of reperfusion therapies. The first goal in mastering stroke diagnosis and treatment is to be able to work fast and efficiently and to start rescue therapies with as little time wasted as possible. Thus much emphasis is placed on shortening the door-to-needle time and the rapidity of reperfusion [1–3]. As a consequence of this pressure, there is often some simplification of the diagnostic workup or abbreviation of imaging sequences in favor of adherence to conventional timeframes for reperfusion therapies. Some further advocate that patient selection criteria for acute reperfusion therapies should be simplified within the traditional window for systemic therapy [4]. Neurological examination should be quick and focused on the presence of disabling symptoms. Ultrasound should be the used for rapid confirmation of the vascular origin of these symptoms and localization of the arterial obstruction. Using cerebrovascular ultrasound in this setting requires superb technical skills and the ability to quickly focus on the key findings supporting or refuting your clinical hypothesis. This book will take you on a journey to reach this level.

Despite the efforts to bring more patients to treatment within the timeframe, still only a minority receive reperfusion therapies. If a patient arrives outside the conventional time window, the sense of urgency is almost always lost, and patients with potentially salvageable or at least partially reversible strokes are not recognized and opportunities are wasted. Every patient is on his or her own clock when it comes to how quickly or slowly they would loose the battle with a thromboembolic occlusion or hypoperfusion. Multimodal brain imaging reveals the heterogeneity of penumbral patterns and ischemic core expansions. The time course of cerebral ischemia is blood-flow dependent and the "time is brain" relationship is not linear [5]. The knowledge that you can gain by mastering the elucidation of the stroke pathogenic mechanism, imaging the residual and collateral flow, prognostication of tissue fate, the ability to manipulate systemic and cerebral hemodynamics, and the assessment of pathophysiological changes in real time will give you a much broader view of how you can devise an appropriate course of action for all patients and, eventually, for many, do something more than advise "take aspirin, go home" or provide just basic care.

In the absence of a better marker, we use the time of symptom onset or time from "last seen normal" as a substitute for the onset of ischemia and timing of occlusion. However, the impact of occlusion and ischemia on the fate of brain tissue is determined and redetermined by several other, often continually changing, environmental factors, both within the brain and throughout the body. In reality, neurological symptoms develop when the collateral flow fails [5] or when the residual flow fails in vessels without further collateral supply. This may not necessarily coincide with the timing of a thrombosis or lodging of an embolus. Pre-existing atheromatous stenoses in the proximal ICA or intracranial vasculature would have been developing over time, allowing for collaterals to develop, while a cardioembolic occlusion suddenly challenges the brain to adapt. The time course of symptomatology and reversibility of the cerebral tissue damage will be different under these circumstances. Progression of the intracranial disease from the M1 MCA stenosis to a complete occlusion may leave such patient with a small stroke while the same location for an abrupt embolic occlusion could leave the patient with atrial fibrillation devastated. While striving to beat the time clock, also remember that "Brain is Flow!": imaging collateral flow and tissue perfusion in general can help you find hemodynamic compromise and search for treatment solutions regardless of the time window [5].

We group patients with heterogeneous stroke mechanisms into specific time frames (i.e. 3, 4.5, 6, 8 hours, etc.) not because of a uniform pathobiological time dependency but because the earlier the patient presents and is treated, the greater the chance that reperfusion therapy will work [6]. This became evident in the thrombolysis clinical trials because most acute ischemic stroke patients have thromboembolic occlusions and could respond to flow-restorative treatments [7]. The illustrative case studies below will address first how to use ultrasound examination in the "time is brain" situation within conventional timeframes for reperfusion.

Case study 2.1

An 82-year-old woman with a past medical history of arterial hypertension and coronary artery disease suddenly developed right-sided weakness and inability to speak, witnessed by her caregiver as she slumped in a chair at an assisted-living facility, 1 hour prior to arrival at the Emergency Department. A prehospital alert was sent and Code Stroke was activated upon her arrival. Her arterial blood pressure was 192/85 mmHg, her ECG in the ambulance showed atrial fibrillation, and she was attached to a portable monitoring system. Oxygen saturation was 99% while on 3 L oxygen via a nasal cannula. Upon brief observation, she was alert and had forced gaze deviation with her head turned to the left. Her right arm did not move in response to a nurse sticking a needle to draw blood and to place the second intravenous access. Her right foot was rotated outward. When an emergency medicine doctor approaches close to her face on the left, she did not answer the question "what is your name?" She was agitated, grabbing the bed side rail with her left hand.

The stroke team moved her stretcher to obtain a noncontrast head CT. CT showed no evidence of hemorrhage, while a hyperdense left M1 MCA sign was present (Figure 2.1).

There was no immediate family available, and an emergency staff member was on the phone to the assisted living facility to find out how to get in touch with her next of kin. Her caregiver also stated over the phone that she was not taking warfarin or any

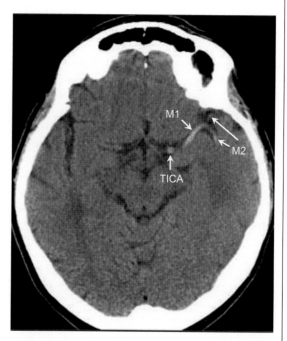

Figure 2.1 Hyperdense left MCA artery sign. M1 and M2 denote the first and second segments of the MCA. TICA, terminal internal carotid artery.

direct thrombin inhibitor and she had a living will that specifically states "no heroic measures and no dependency on artificial life sustaining measures." The phone number for her son rang into a voicemail.

1. What is the diagnosis?

An acute and severe ischemic stroke.

2. Is the patient a candidate for intravenous tPA?

Yes (even though she was an octogenarian with the total NIHSS score of 27 points). There is no upper age limit nor too low or too high NIHSS score within 3 hours of symptom onset according to the National Institutes of Neurological Disorders and Stroke (NINDS) rt-PA Stroke Study criteria [8].

3. Do you need to obtain consent?

Given that she was aphasic, and her son could not be reached, you needed a second attending physician to concur that the standard of care systemic tPA therapy was appropriate and can be given in her case without violation of the FDA label, given the information available at the time.

4. Is this patient going to respond to systemic tPA?

Patients with severe strokes and advanced age are less likely to recover compared to younger patients and those with less severe strokes [9]. However, they did fare better than patients with similar age and stroke severity in the placebo arm of the NINDS–rt-PA Stroke Study and in a subsequent re-analysis of the acute stroke trials database in the Virtual International Stroke Trials Archive (VISTA) [10]. Furthermore, patients with proximal arterial occlusions are less likely to recanalize with systemic tPA therapy alone [11]. Given her advanced age and current limitations with endovascular access in this age group, systemic tPA is the only feasible reperfusion option for this patient.

As you can see from a brief neurological observation and image interpretation, one can obtain enough information to justify taking the risks of tPA treatment in view of the devastating nature of her stroke. Two attending-level physicians concurred in this assessment.

5. When should tPA be given?

Systemic tPA should be started as soon as possible. No additional imaging (besides noncontrast head CT) is required within the approved time window for tPA because only noncontrast head CT was used in the NINDS–rt-PA Stroke Study to rule out intracerebral hemorrhage and no vascular or multimodal imaging was available for emergent workup nor was it required in the pivotal trial.

6. Is this patient ready to get tPA?

Not until her arterial blood pressure is below 185/110 mmHg before tPA bolus and below 180/105 mmHg thereafter. If BP still requires correction, we prefer starting our candidates for thrombolysis on intravenous infusion of nicardipine (a short-acting calcium channel blocker) because not only do you have to lower BP before tPA, it should also remain under tight control during the subsequent hospital stay (of course, the transition to oral medicines should occur as soon as feasible). Nicardipine infusion was started at the rate of 5 mg/h and her BP reduced to 163/85 mmHg. Intravenous tPA was started at 10% bolus (0.9 mg/kg, maximum dose 90 mg) and 90% continuous infusion over 1 hour.

7. Is there a role for vascular imaging before tPA bolus?

Yes, as our knowledge of how tPA works or fails has grown since the NINDS–rt-PA Stroke Study as well as our ability to rapidly image cerebral vasculature with CT-angiography (CTA), focused MRI protocols, and ultrasound. We now know that intravenous tPA breaks up distal thrombi more efficiently, with complete recanalization rates of approximately 40% for the M2 MCA, 20% for M1 MCA, and less than 10% for the terminal ICA [11]. Thus, knowledge of the occlusion location before tPA bolus can expedite additional decision making, such as consideration of adjuvant therapies to augment activity of tPA or endovascular reperfusion procedures.

This patient had noncontrast head CT findings also suspect for hyperdense left terminal ICA (TICA) that can be seen as a "dot" sign (Figure 2.1). The finding of an acute TICA occlusion implies a much worse prognosis and would be helpful in discussions with her family about subsequent goals of care. TCD could be a quick way to confirm or refute the presence of TICA occlusion versus a calcified vessel on CT scan. A blunted left M1 MCA signal and normal systolic flow acceleration in the left A1 anterior cerebral artery (ACA) segment (Figure 2.2) are findings indicative of a proximal MCA occlusion as opposed to a "T"-type terminal ICA occlusion when both M1 and A1 are affected. These TCD findings may not completely rule out the "L" type of the terminal ICA occlusion where a thrombus extends into the M1

(Continued)

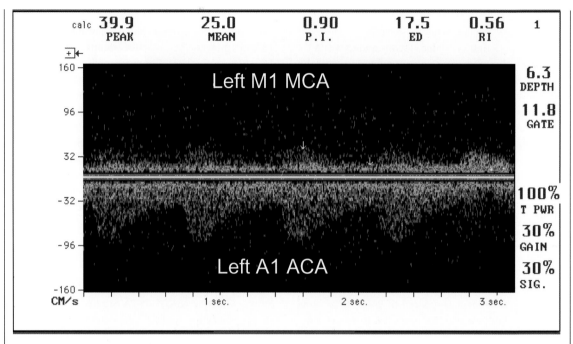

| calc **39.9** | **25.0** | **0.90** | **17.5** | **0.56** | 1 |
| PEAK | MEAN | P.I. | ED | RI | |

Left M1 MCA

Left A1 ACA

6.3 DEPTH

11.8 GATE

100% T PWR

30% GAIN

30% SIG.

Figure 2.2 Spectral waveform findings indicative of the right MCA occlusion. The blunted MCA signal above the baseline has a flattened shape, while the ACA signal below has good systolic flow acceleration and velocity higher than the unilateral MCA.

MCA from the terminal ICA. Nonetheless, these detectable residual flow signals show that an acute occlusion is present and is not complete. Complete occlusions present with no detectable flow signals while detectable residual flow signals predict increased likelihood of early recanalization during systemic tPA therapy [12].

At a comprehensive stroke center level, carotid duplex and transcranial Doppler should be routinely available [13]. Ultrasound, particularly TCD, offers noninvasive repeatable testing of the proximal cerebral vessels in real time. TCD and carotid duplex have high yield in detection of lesions amenable to intervention in the acute phase of cerebral ischemia [14]. They offer information complimentary to the advanced multimodal imaging such as CT/CTA/CTP and MRI/MRA because these tests are often done only once with the main limitations being exposure to X rays and patient tolerability. Ultrasound monitoring of the intracranial lesions and flow dynamics and direct visualization of plaque and thrombi on the neck are the key advantages that a skilled opera-

tor and knowledgeable interpreter can bring to the emergency room.

The NIHSS is predictive of thrombus presence, that is an occlusion is present in 100% of acute patients with NIHSS ≥15, and in 70% of those with NIHSS ≥9 points [15]. However, NIHSS is nonspecific to the thrombus location(s). Furthermore, in the mild NIHSS range (<6 points) is not a guarantee that there is no M1 MCA, tandem ICA/MCA occlusion, or a lesion in the posterior circulation. Finally, a complete neurological deficit resolution should not be taken as evidence for complete recanalization. Such improvement simply means that the patient has "recoverable" brain and either some degree of recanalization occurred or collateral flow compensated for the persisting lesion. Ultrasound tests at the bedside can rapidly localize occlusion(s), detect collaterals and ongoing cerebral vessel embolization, and give clues to the underlying mechanism of stroke, recovery, or lack there of. Patients who are not clinically improving and recanalizing during tPA infusion have approximately 80% chance of poor long-term outcomes (i.e.

modified Rankin scores 2–6) and these patients are now increasingly being considered tPA "failures": ultrasound detection of the persisting arterial occlusion can be used as further evidence in support of additional aggressive measures [16]. Continuous ultrasound monitoring during and shortly after tPA infusion enables us to not "fly in the dark."

Returning to our patient, she had no recanalization at the end of tPA infusion on TCD and no neurological improvement over the subsequent 24 hours. Repeat brain imaging showed an evolving large left MCA infarct without hemorrhagic transformation. A family meeting was held the next day and they opted for palliative care.

Case study 2.2

A 56-year-old woman with history of hypertension was found on the floor at home, and was brought to our emergency room 45 minutes after last seen normal (for additional discussion see reference [17]). She had left hemiplegia and dysarthria. While neglecting her problems on the left side of the body, her chief complaint was bilateral ear and midsternal chest pain.

On examination, her blood pressure was 108/56 mmHg with a heart rate of 51. Her heart sounds were regular without any murmurs and peripheral arterial pulses were symmetric. She was awake, and her speech was slow and dysarthric. Comprehension and naming were intact. She had left hemineglect and her eyes deviated to the right. She had left hemianopia, left hemiparesis, and left hemisensory loss. The total NIHSS score was 16 points. A noncontrast CT scan of the head was normal.

1. What is the diagnosis?

An acute ischemic stroke, although concurrent myocardial ischemia or aortic dissection should also be suspected.

Her ECG showed sinus bradycardia without any changes suggestive of myocardial ischemia, and her laboratory studies, including creatinine kinase and troponin, were normal. Chest X ray was normal without pulmonary edema or mediastinal widening to suggest aortic dissection. Urgent transthoracic echocardiography (TTE) was performed in the emergency room due to suspicion of cardiac ischemia or aortic dissection. TTE showed no wall motion abnormalities, pericardial effusion, tamponade, or aortic insufficiency.

2. Can this patient be treated with tPA?

If this patient is having a stroke and myocardial ischemia at the same time, intravenous tPA will be helping to dissolve both cerebral and coronary thrombi. If there is an aortic dissection, intravenous tPA should not be given.

Chest CTA was considered, but not done immediately because it is not part of a routine pre-tPA workup within the window for thrombolysis and the need to treat the patient for stroke without delay. Intravenous tPA was started at 150 minutes after stroke onset.

TCD showed waveform changes consistent with the right MCA occlusion (Figure 2.3) and indirect evidence of a hemodynamically significant lesion in the proximal ICA, that is either an occlusion or a stenosis that causes perfusion pressure drop in the distal vasculature and induces recruitment of collaterals. Carotid duplex examination with a portable scanner showed a proximal right common carotid artery (CCA) and left CCA occlusions with thrombi (Figure 2.4).

3. How common are tandem MCA/ICA thromboembolic or atherothrombotic occlusions in acute stroke patients who are candidates for intravenous tPA?

In the Combined Lysis of Thrombus in Brain Ischemia using Transcranial Ultrasound and Systemic tPA (CLOTBUST) trial approximately one-third of patients presenting with acute M1 or M2 MCA occlusions also had a thrombus in the ICA or severe atheromatous stenosis [18]. However, none had a lesion in the CCA in this trial and CCAs are rarely affected by a significant atheromatous stenosis.

(Continued)

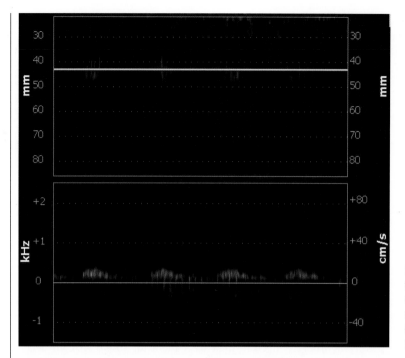

Figure 2.3 Minimal flow signal in the distal M1 MCA consistent with its occlusion. Systolic spikes and absent diastolic flow at the depth of 45 mm (trans-temporal insonation with TCD) indicate distal M1 MCA occlusion.

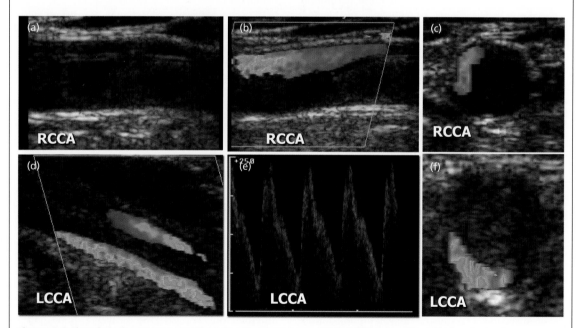

Figure 2.4 Thrombi in the common carotid arteries. Upper row images labeled RCCA show B-mode (**a**) and color flow (**b**, **c**) findings in the right CCA: two longitudinal projections and one transverse view. Bottom row images labeled LCCA show a longitudinal view of the residual lumen in the left CCA and flow in the jugular vein above moving in the opposite direction (**d**); spectrogram of a stenotic flow signal in the left CCA (**e**), and a transverse view of the intraluminal thrombus and the residual lumen in the left CCA (**f**).

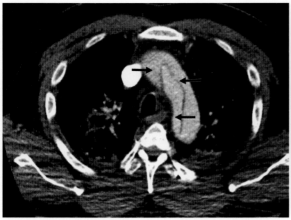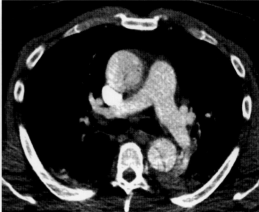

Figure 2.5 Chest CT-angiography showing aortic dissection.

B-mode findings of a thrombus in both CCAs are unusual for an acute stroke presentation. Therefore the reasons for thrombi presence in the CCAs should be ascertained. Sometimes an embolus originating from the heart gets trapped proximal to a stenosis, or thrombosis could have descended down from it or created a stagnant segment of the vessel with reverberating (oscillating) or minimal blood flow signals mimicking occlusion. The worst scenario, however, is an aortic dissection extending to the right and left common carotid arteries up to its bifurcations, a feature that differentiates the aortic dissection from the distal ICA when the dissection travels down the vessel but stops at the bulb and does not affect the CCA.

The aortic dissection can be further suspected from an intraluminal intimal flap that can be visualized within the proximal CCA with or without a thrombus. When CCA thrombus was found on ultrasound after tPA infusion started, tPA was stopped, and the patient was taken for urgent chest CTA that revealed type A thoracic aortic dissection (Figure 2.5).

4. What should be done next?

Intravenous tPA infusion was stopped due to a possibility that systemic thrombolysis may worsen the dissection, and cardiovascular surgery needed to be urgently notified.

5. What could have been done differently in this case?

Sternal chest pain in an acute stroke patient (when known from the start and with no evidence for myocardial ischemia) should prompt chest CTA to be done immediately after CT of the head to rule out aortic dissection. Carotid duplex could have been performed faster and before tPA bolus to look at both proximal CCAs for flaps or thrombi. Low blood pressures in the absence of myocardial ischemia should further have raised the suspicion because arterial blood pressures tend to be high with acute stroke presentations. Finally, ringing in the ear has not been reported for aortic dissections but ear pain (as referred facial pain) has been reported for the ICA dissections [19].

Working with the team of cardiovascular surgeons led by Hazim Safi allowed the hospital's urgent aortic repair protocol to be activated. The patient underwent emergent surgical repair of the dissection with a Dacron woven tube graft. Intraoperative transesophageal echocardiography (TEE) visualized the ascending aortic dissection and moderate aortic insufficiency. Hypothermic arrest and retrograde perfusion of the brain for 28 minutes was monitored with TCD that showed low-resistance blood flow signals in the MCA that were reversed in direction, that is blood was flowing from M2 segments into M1 and TICA (Figure 2.6). This low-resistance reversed flow

(Continued)

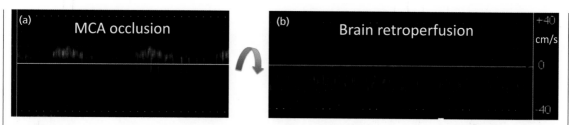

Figure 2.6 Flow reversal in the affected MCA during brain retroperfusion. (**a**) Spectrogram shows an antegrade minimal high-resistance flow signal in the right MCA before treatment. (**b**) Spectrogram obtained at the same depth through the temporal bone insonation during urgent repair of the aorta when brain retroperfusion was initiated during profound hypothermic cardiac arrest.

indicates possible retrograde flushing of the MCA thrombus into the carotid and brachicephalic vessels.

The inhospital course was complicated by arrhythmias, acute renal failure, and pneumonia. Follow-up MRI of the brain showed the right MCA infarction while intracranial MRA was normal. At 3 months, her stroke symptoms had not improved significantly and she had a modified Rankin score of 4 (moderately severe disability) and Glasgow Outcome Scale of 3 (severe disability) [17]. However, she has survived the likely fatal event. Of note, both acute interventions could have been withheld according to the "finding the reasons not to treat" philosophy.

There are no answers in the evidence-based literature on how to reverse or reduce the disability in a patient in this situation. However, the knowledge of the mechanism and hemodynamic changes allowed

at least an attempt to rescue the vessels with the goal of restoring blood flow to the brain. Subsequent deployment of TCD monitoring during urgent repairs of the aortic type A dissections allowed cardiovascular surgeons at UT-Houston and Zsolt Garami, MD to demonstrate that these repairs can be done safely even if the dissection is complicated by stroke and that TCD monitoring and correction of brain malperfusion reduces the temporary neurological symptomatology that is common with these procedures [20, 21]. Perhaps, these extremely severe and complex cases should stimulate research into treatment decisions that are based on real-time pathophysiological assessments in acute ischemic stroke. Meanwhile, most decisions in acute setting still hinge on often one-time snap-shot images in the consideration of an intervention.

Case study 2.3

A 65-year-old white man with a past medical history of previous myocardial infarction, hypertension, and smoking presented to the emergency room 90 minutes after sudden onset of the left-sided weakness. On examination, he was alert, oriented, and followed commands. He had a partial gaze preference and left sided hemiparesis (arm > leg) with a total NIHSS score of 5 points. A noncontrast CT showed hyperdense distal right MCA with no early ischemic changes in brain tissue, with an ASPECTS score of 10 points. Risks of standard intravenous tPA therapy were explained to the patient and he agreed to receive this. A tPA bolus was given at 122 minutes after stroke onset. At the end of tPA infusion, his NIHSS score was 2 points.

1. Was the patient a good candidate for systemic tPA?

Yes, patients with moderate stroke severity respond to tPA better than those with severe strokes; however, the NINDS–rt-PA Stroke Study was not powered to answer if a subgroup of patients with NIHSS 0–5 benefits more than placebo [22]. Furthermore, the NIHSS score "favors" the left MCA symptoms and thus in reality his stroke may have been more severe. He had cortical symptoms and a larger area of the brain may have been affected. Nonetheless, early reduction in the NIHSS score during treatment is encouraging.

2. At approximately 180 minutes from onset, his remaining deficit included partial gaze preference

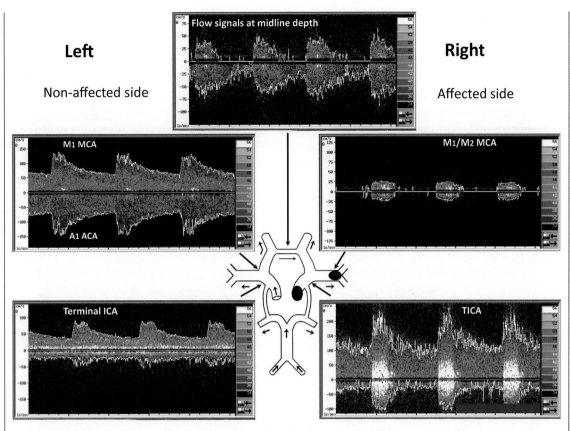

Figure 2.7 Spectral TCD findings of a tandem MCA/ICA obstruction in a patient receiving systemic tPA therapy.

that he can overcome to command, and he did not recognize the doctor touching his left side on double simultaneous stimulation. Can this remaining deficit cause disability?

Yes, patients with neglect or inattention may not return to their prior activities safely, and may not realize the full potential of rehabilitation [23].

3. Should additional reperfusion procedures be considered?

This is an area of uncertainty because endovascular interventions carry their own risk of complications, including symptomatic intracerebral hemorrhage, which could make this patient worse. Early clinical improvement with intravenous tPA should also be viewed as a good prognostic sign and, in the absence of clear efficacy of endovascular procedures to reverse stroke symptoms, these procedures should be reserved for patients with clearly disabling

remaining deficits, no neurological improvement, or with worsening.

4. Is there a role for ultrasound in this patient?

Ultrasound can be used in his case to determine the following:

(a) if complete recanalization of the MCA has indeed occurred;

(b) if there is a persistent distal MCA obstruction;

(c) if there is a lesion in the ICA (artery-to-artery embolization with pre-existing stenosis or embolus fragmentation).

A single-channel TCD showed a minimal mid-M1 flow signal at a depth of 50 mm (Figure 2.7), positive diastolic flow in the proximal MCA, and a stenotic flow signal with harsh systolic bruits at the depths of the terminal ICA, posterior communicating, and posterior cerebral arteries.

(Continued)

No flow signals were obtained from the right siphon and ophthalmic artery through the transorbital window. On the contralateral side, TCD showed flow diversion to the ACA (flow velocities in the left MCA were less than in the left ACA and the proportion of the end diastolic flow in the ACA was greater than in the unilateral MCA, consistent with lesser resistance to flow).

TCD findings were interpreted as follows:

(a) An acute right M1–M2 subdivision occlusion with patent proximal right M1 MCA segment at the origin of perforating vessels; and

(b) A hemodynamically significant, possibly acute, right ICA obstruction likely extending from the neck.

(c) Functioning collateral channels, including the left-to-right anterior cross-filling via the anterior communicating artery and from the posterior to anterior circulation via the right posterior communicating artery.

5. What is the significance of these findings for patient management?

Despite early neurological improvement, recanalization was incomplete and this patient was at risk of worsening. After tPA infusion is completed, tPA half-life is short and if a thrombogenic surface exists, it may result in re-occlusion or re-embolization. Furthermore, TCD points to the existence of a tandem lesion in the ICA that is hemodynamically significant. If this patient worsened neurologically within the next few hours, he may still have been within the window for intra-arterial deployment of a thrombectomy device. Knowledge of whether there is an embolus or atherothrombosis in the ICA could help endovascular specialists to plan the procedure accordingly. Carotid duplex can quickly determine the presence of an atherosclerotic plaque or intraluminal thrombus (see examples in Chapter 1). Finally, the proximal right ICA occlusion may be acute or chronic, and duplex criteria for differentiation will be discussed in subsequent chapters.

This information helped the team to be prepared for deterioration and have an action plan. Angiography also showed a complete proximal ICA occlusion at the bulb and no intervention was performed because no neurological worsening had occurred. Repeat CT at 20 hours after stroke onset showed no hemorrhagic transformation or hypoattenuation in the right MCA territory. Repeat TCD at 48 hours showed complete distal MCA recanalization and sustained intracranial collateral flow compensating for ICA occlusion. His modified Rankin score at 3 months was 0.

This case illustrates the fact that the presence of an ICA occlusion should not be viewed as an insurmountable lesion location for tPA to benefit acute stroke patients. In a large multicenter study, patients with ICA occlusions who were treated with i.v. tPA within conventional time windows did better than matched case controls [24]. Systemic tPA works in those patients mostly by recanalizing the distal tip of the thrombus or just a tandem MCA thromboembolic occlusion. Collaterals, if recruited timely, help maintain brain perfusion despite persistence of the ICA occlusion after treatment.

References

1. Meretoja A, Strbian D, Mustanoja S, *et al.* Reducing in-hospital delay to 20 minutes in stroke thrombolysis. *Neurology* 2012; **79**: 306–13.

2. Alexandrov AV, Schelliger PD, Saqqur M, *et al.* Reperfusion and clinical outcomes in Penumbra vs. systemic tissue plasminogen activator clinical trials. *Intl J Stroke* 2011; **6**: 118–22.

3. Khatri P, Abruzzo T, Yeatts SD, *et al.* IMS I and II Investigators. Good clinical outcome after ischemic stroke with successful revascularization is time-dependent. *Neurology* 2009; **73**: 1066–72.

4. Tong DC. Avoiding thrombolysis in patients with mild stroke: is it SMART? *Stroke* 2012; **43**: 625–6.

5. Liebeskind DS. Time is brain – revisited. In: Liebeskind DS (ed). *Diagnostic Strategies in Cerebral Ischemia.* Oxford: Clinical Publishing, 2011, pp. 13–22.

6. Hacke W, Donnan G, Fieschi C, *et al.* Association of outcome with early stroke treatment: pooled analysis of ATLANTIS, ECASS, and NINDS rt-PA stroke trials. *Lancet* 2004; **363**: 768–74.

7. Rha JH, Saver JL. The impact of recanalization on ischemic stroke outcome: a meta-analysis. *Stroke* 2007; **38**: 967–73.

8. The National Institutes of Neurological Disorders and Stroke rt-PA Stroke Study Group. Tissue plasminogen

activator for acute ischemic stroke. *N Engl J Med* 1995; **333**: 1581–7.

9. Chen CI, Iguchi Y, Grotta JC, *et al.* Intravenous TPA for very old stroke patients. *Eur Neurol* 2005; **54**: 140–4.

10. Frank B, Grotta JC, Alexandrov AV, *et al.* for the VISTA Collaborators. Thrombolysis in stroke despite contraindications or warnings? *Stroke* 2013; in press.

11. Saqqur M, Uchino K, Demchuk AM, *et al.* Site of arterial occlusion identified by transcranial Doppler (TCD) predicts the response to intravenous thrombolysis for stroke. *Stroke* 2007; **38**: 948–54.

12. Labiche LA, Malkoff M, Alexandrov AV. Residual flow signals predict complete recanalization in stroke patients treated with TPA. *J Neuroimaging* 2003; **13**: 28–33.

13. Alberts MJ, Latchaw RE, Selman WR, *et al.* for the Brain Attack Coalition. Recommendations for comprehensive stroke centers: a consensus statement from the brain attack coalition. *Stroke* 2005; **36**: 1597–618.

14. Chernyshev OY, Garami Z, Calleja S, *et al.* The yield and accuracy of urgent combined carotid-transcranial ultrasound testing in acute cerebral ischemia. *Stroke* 2005; **36**: 32–7.

15. Lewandowski CA, Frankel M, Tomsick TA, *et al.* Combined intravenous and intra-arterial r-TPA versus intra-arterial therapy of acute ischemic stroke: Emergency Management of Stroke (EMS) Bridging Trial. *Stroke* 1999; **30**: 2598–605.

16. Labiche LA, Al-Senani F, Wojner AW, *et al.* Is the benefit of early recanalization sustained at 3 months? A prospective cohort study. *Stroke* 2003; **34**: 695–8.

17. Uchino K, Estrera A, Calleja S, *et al.* Aortic dissection presenting as an acute ischemic stroke for thrombolysis. *J Neuroimaging* 2005; **15**: 281–3.

18. Alexandrov AV, Molina CA, Grotta JC, *et al.* Ultrasound-enhanced systemic thrombolysis for acute ischemic stroke. *N Engl J Med* 2004; **351**: 2170–8.

19. Silbert PL, Mokri B, Schievink WI. Headache and neck pain in spontaneous internal carotid and vertebral artery dissections. *Neurology* 1995; **45**: 1517–22.

20. Estrera AL, Garami Z, Miller CC, *et al.* Acute type A aortic dissection complicated by stroke: can immediate repair be performed safely? *J Thorac Cardiovasc Surg* 2006; **132**: 1404–8.

21. Estrera AL, Garami Z, Miller CC 3rd, *et al.* Cerebral monitoring with transcranial Doppler ultrasonography improves neurologic outcome during repairs of acute type A aortic dissection. *J Thorac Cardiovasc Surg* 2005; **129**: 277–85.

22. Ingall TJ, O'Fallon WM, Asplund K, *et al.* Findings from the reanalysis of the NINDS tissue plasminogen activator for acute ischemic stroke treatment trial. *Stroke* 2004; **35**: 2418–24.

23. Lyden PD (ed). *Thrombolytic Therapy for Acute Stroke*, 2nd edn. Totowa: Humana Press, 2005.

24. Paciaroni M, Balucani C, Agnelli G, *et al.* Systemic thrombolysis in patients with acute ischemic stroke and internal carotid artery occlusion: the ICARO study. *Stroke* 2012; **43**: 125–30.

3 The Power of Observation

"Thinking is more interesting than knowing, but less interesting than looking."

Johann Wolfgang von Goethe

Let's now look into a broader scope of stroke-related problems that often lie outside the comfort zone of established evidence. For instance, the pivotal clinical trials of systemic tPA such as the NINDS–rt-PA Stroke Study and European Cooperative Acute Stroke Study (ECASS) trials showed that tPA helped more patients recover at 3 months after ischemic stroke but did not show the so-called Lazarus effect during and shortly after treatment [1, 2]. In the NINDS–rt-PA Stroke Study there was no difference in reduction of the NIHSS scores at 2 hours after tPA bolus compared to placebo [1]. Unlike myocardial infarction, when chest pain goes away and electrocardiographic activity improves with successful thrombolysis, intravenous tPA for stroke did not produce immediate neurological symptom alleviation in pivotal trials.

The debate about how and if tPA works prompted our group to depart from the snap-shot assessments of parenchyma and perfusion to real-time monitoring of the residual flow around a thrombus and changes in cerebral hemodynamics [3]. Faced by the challenge to demonstrate an acute occlusion in patients presenting within the timeframe for intravenous tPA [4], we also were interested to see when tPA works or fails. The following Case studies 3.1 through 3.3 were the first experiences in monitoring the residual flow signals, reperfusion, and re-occlusion during intravenous tPA therapy [5–7]. These observations led to a series of studies and clinical trials that laid the foundation for clinical sonothrombolysis [8], or the way to amplify the systemic ability of tPA to break up thromboembolic occlusions. Observations of re-occlusion and persisting arterial occlusion opened the quest for therapies adjuvant to tPA [9], and provided some rationale of why certain patients should be considered for additional endovascular reperfusion procedures.

Neurovascular Examination: The Rapid Evaluation of Stroke Patients Using Ultrasound Waveform Interpretation, First Edition.
Andrei V. Alexandrov.
© 2013 Andrei V. Alexandrov. Published 2013 by Blackwell Publishing Ltd.

Case study 3.1 Dramatic neurological recovery during thrombolysis

While at work at 2:50 PM, an 85-year-old right-handed woman suddenly became mute and weak on her right side (for additional discussion, see reference [5]). She arrived at the hospital at 3:32 PM, and head CT at 3:50 PM showed no hemorrhage and no early ischemic changes. Her total NIHSS score was 12 points. Noncontrast head CT showed questionable sulcal effacement in the left MCA cortex with total ASPECTS score of 9 points. At 4: 05 PM, TCD showed a minimal flow signal in the left middle cerebral artery (MCA) (Figure 3.1). The residual flow signals in the MCA were monitored at a constant angle with use of a 2-MHz transducer mounted on a head frame.

Treatment with t-PA (0.9 mg per kg of body weight intravenously, 10% bolus) was initiated with bolus at 4:12 PM. At 4:46 PM, a sudden embolic signal was heard (arrow in Figure 3.1), followed by the sudden restoration of a normal waveform, suggesting complete reperfusion of the MCA. Five minutes later, the

patient began to regain strength in her right arm. At 5 PM she began smiling, laughing, and using single words to speak with family members. By 5:10 PM she could speak in full sentences and had no residual motor weakness. She had only mild difficulties with comprehension and repetition when she was assessed at 5:26 PM. Total NIHSS score was 2 points.

By the next morning she had no residual deficit (NIHSS 0). Aspirin 325 mg daily was initiated 24 hours after the infusion of t-PA. The patient was sent home with advice to continue taking aspirin, and she returned to work full time 6 days after the event. She was placed on 30-day heart monitor/ event detector but no atrial fibrillation was confirmed. She remained free of neurologic symptoms 4 months later.

While at University of Texas–Houston Medical School in late 1990s, our team observed and reported more similar recoveries [10]. Patti Bratina, RN the clinical trial coordinator previously responsible for the NINDS–rt-PA Study at UT, made an observation

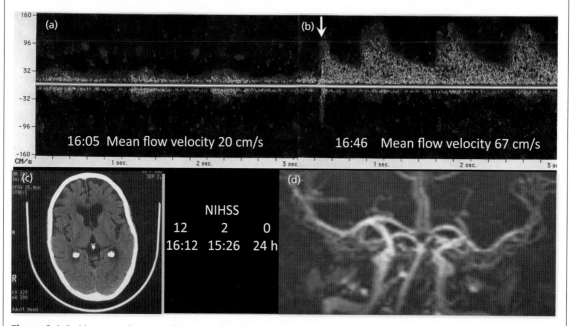

Figure 3.1 Sudden recanalization and dramatic clinical recovery during intravenous tPA infusion. (**a**) A spectrogram of the residual flow signal in the obstructed left MCA before tPA bolus; (**b**) an embolic signal (arrow) and sudden restoration of a low-resistance normal waveform in the left MCA. (**c**) Pretreatment noncontrast head CT scan; (**d**) intracranial MRA showing normal patency of the left MCA post-treatment.

at rounds that since sonographers started to show up in the Emergency Department to monitor thrombolytic therapy, more patients started to recover during treatment, and this was something she has not seen before. In fact, there were no differences in the NIHSS scores between placebo and tPA treated patients at 2 hours after tPA bolus [1]. The difference only became detectable at 24 hours but not by the prespecified early neurological end-point by 4 NIHSS points or more [11]. More patients receiving tPA had 5+ NIHSS points improvement at 24 hours compared to placebo [1, 11]. This observation of a dramatic neurological recovery during treatment and discussion with team members sparkled a series of clinical studies of sonothrombolysis to amplify the only approved therapy to reverse ischemic stroke.

Case study 3.2 Real-time recanalization and reperfusion process

A 56-year-old man suddenly developed the right-sided weakness and inability to talk (for additional discussion, see reference [6]). He presented to the Emergency Department in the timeframe to receive systemic tPA and had no known contraindications. His total NIHSS score was 23 points and an occlusion of the left M1 MCA on TCD (minimal systolic signal at the depth of 53 mm). A helmet was placed for monitoring the residual flow signals during tPA treatment in real time at a steady angle of insonation.

At the initiation of rtPA treatment, only minimal flow signals were visualized (systolic spikes with absent diastolic flow, Figure 3.2, Frame 1) indicating an acute M1 MCA occlusion. The MCA flow signals started to improve 30 minutes later during tPA infusion (Figure 3.2, Frames 2, 3). Microembolic signals were heard as chirping sounds with unidirectional appearance on screen (white arrow, Figure 3.2, Frame 2) consistent with the beginning of thrombus breakdown and washout. A brief period of a stenotic signal was seen (Figure 3.2, Frame 4) representing early reperfusion with a residual stenosis. This was rapidly followed by appearance of a hyperemic low-resistance flow (above age-expected mean flow velocities and disproportionately high diastolic flow velocities, Figure 3.2, Frames 5, 6) indicating complete MCA recanalization at 36 minutes after initiating rtPA infusion.

Although at that time we were still fascinated by the ability of TCD to demonstrate recanalization in real time, this case also gave us an insight into how hemorrhagic transformation can occur after systemic tPA infusion. At 5–7 hours from symptom onset,

the patient became drowsy, stopped following commands, and urgent head CT scan showed parenchymal hemorrhage type 2 with mass effect. The patient expired next day.

A retrospective analysis of this case during our regular morbidity and mortality conference showed that this massive hemorrhage occurred after early and complete MCA recanalization with arterial blood pressures not exceeding 180/105 mmHg, as required by the standard tPA protocol. The missing link was the hyperemic nature of this reperfusion evident from a very low resistance to flow (high diastolic velocity on TCD). This finding indicates that brain cannot regulate the incoming flow well with higher pressures delivering more flow volume, and perhaps the blood pressure range up to 180 systolic and 105 mmHg diastolic is too generous for those who reperfuse completely.

Over subsequent years, we started to pay even closer attention to BP management and the following algorithm was developed:
1. bring BP below 185/105 mmHg before tPA bolus;
2. during tPA infusion and thereafter BP should under no circumstances exceed 180/105 mmHg;
3. ideally, we try to keep BP in 140–160 systolic and under 80 mmHg diastolic;
4. once complete reperfusion is achieved, our BP goals should be below 140/80 mmHg;
5. patients with persisting arterial occlusions beyond 2 hours of tPA bolus are at higher risk of hemorrhagic complications compared to those who recanalize early [12], and this group of patients should be watched more closely for late reperfusion.

(Continued)

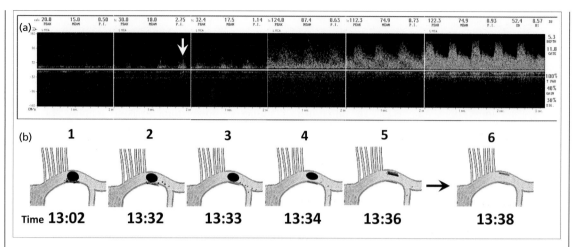

Figure 3.2 Stepwise recanalization of the M1 MCA during intravenous tPA infusion. (**a**) TCD recordings were obtained via the transtemporal approach at the depth of 53 mm with a 11.8 mm gate of insonation using single channel 2 MHz TCD. (**b**) Graphic showing our interpretation of the waveform findings and presumed thrombus location in the MCA main stem. Real time (military) is provided below. **Frame 1** A minimal flow signal in the proximal MCA at the time of intravenous rtPA bolus (13: 02). No changes were seen for the next 30 minutes of continuous intravenous rtPA infusion. **Frames 2 and 3** At 13: 32, the beginning of recanalization was noticed with increasing velocities and microembolic signals (arrow). **Frame 4** Continuing recanalization with a turbulent stenotic signal and audible chirping components suggesting continuing thrombus dissolution. **Frame 5** Hyperemic flow with velocities elevated above age-expected values and relatively low pulsatility (Gosling pulsatility index 0.73) indicating distal vasodilation. Note some evidence of persisting turbulence ("feathering" of the waveform along the top frequencies during the cardiac cycle). **Frame 6** Hyperemic flow with velocities elevated above age-expected values and normal pulsatility (Gosling pulsatility index 0.93) showing a proximal MCA reperfusion with distal vasomotor response. Complete MCA recanalization with low-resistance distal reperfusion was diagnosed at 36 minutes after tPA bolus.

This is the area where more data on reperfusion and BP management are becoming available [13]. Skeptics of acute blood pressure lowering may bring up a caveat that in most ischemic stroke patients BP decreases over time on its own and this is presumed to occur with delayed recanalization or infarct stabilization. However, the rationale to treat blood pressure in acute ischemic stroke existed even before the thrombolytic era [14]. With emphasis on thrombolysis, BP management becomes of paramount importance. Perhaps those who recanalize late (>2 hours after tPA bolus) at blood pressures towards the high end of allowed range or in violation of this safety limit are at the highest risk of symptomatic ICH (sICH).

Fortunately, as our experience with systemic thrombolysis grows, the rates of sICH at busy centers fall mostly under 3% compared to 6.4% in the pivotal NINDS–rt-PA study [15]. Nonetheless, this subject still deserves vigilant attention from both trainees and experienced vascular neurologists [16]. We now also have preliminary observations with TCD monitoring of endovascular reperfusion procedures that hyperemia after successful thrombectomy can occur [17] and we manage BP more aggressively in those patients, that is setting the goal to reach <140/80 mmHg as soon as possible. Ultrasound monitoring can provide fast and objective information about hyperemia because it is able to compare the affected and nonaffected vessels simultaneously. This information is complimentary to catheter angiography and ultrasound can pick up these events before hyperemic reperfusion becomes obvious on the angiogram, CT, or clinically.

Case study 3.3 Arterial re-occlusion

A 42-year-old right handed woman was seen 80 minutes after the acute onset of right-sided weakness and inability to speak (for additional discussion, see reference [7]). Her past medial history included smoking, noninsulin-dependent diabetes, and peripheral vascular disease with bilateral femoral–popliteal bypasses with no history of cardiac or cerebral ischemia, and the patient was not on any antiplatelet regimen. On exam she had right-sided hemiplegia, global aphasia, eye deviation to the left, and a right homonymous hemianopsia (her total NIHSS score was 24 points).

We started evaluating her intracranial vasculature with TCD in parallel with the neurological examination and at 90 minutes from symptom onset she had high-resistance waveforms, indicating a proximal M1 MCA and A1 anterior cerebral artery (ACA) occlusions (Figure 3.3, Frame 1) followed by rapid progression to a terminal internal carotid artery (ICA) occlusion (Figure 3.3, Frame 2). Within 5 minutes, she became drowsy and her total NIHSS score increased to 26 points. Head CT showed a hyperdense left MCA sign and no hemorrhage. Intravenous tPA was started at 120 minutes from

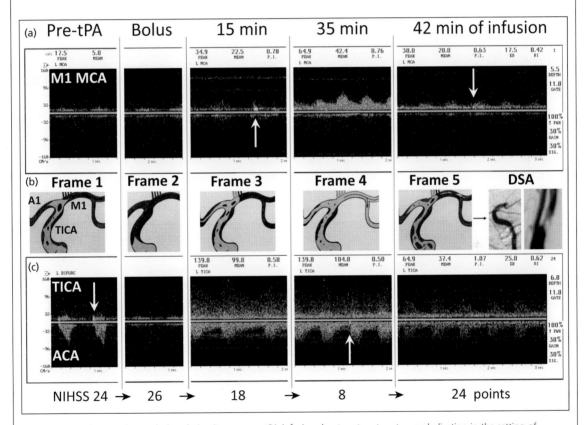

Figure 3.3 Early arterial re-occlusion during intravenous tPA infusion due to artery-to-artery embolization in the setting of large-vessel atherothrombosis. Time-corresponding spectral waveforms in the (**a**) M1 MCA and (**c**) TICA bifurcations. (**b**) Drawings indicate our interpretation of the Doppler findings. Corresponding NIHSS scores are provided below. Catheter angiography was done at the end of tPA infusion showing a severe (>70% NASCET) ulcerated atheromatous stenosis in the proximal ICA and the terminal ICA occlusion above the knee of the ICA siphon.

(Continued)

symptom onset using a standard dose of 0.9 mg/kg (10% bolus, 90% infusion over 1 hour, maximum dose 90 mg).

At 10 minutes after tPA bolus, TCD showed terminal ICA recanalization with appearance of positive diastolic flow in the A1 ACA, followed shortly by improvement in her level of consciousness. Cartoon inserts in Figure 3.3b demonstrate our interpretation of the waveforms obtained from the branches of the TICA. At 15 minutes of infusion, high-intensity transient embolic signals were detected in the M1 MCA accompanied with proximal M1 segment recanalization and resumption of positive diastolic flow at the insonation depths (55–68 mm) suggestive of reperfusion of the M1 MCA origin and at least some of her perforating arteries (Figure 3.3, Frame 3). Clinically, her right leg began to move followed by antigravity strength in the distal arm and improved facial weakness (total NIHSS score 18).

TCD showed a continuing recanalization of the A1 ACA at 20 minutes, followed by resolution of her gaze preference and continued improvement in her right-sided weakness by 30 minutes (total NIHSS score 15). At 35 minutes, she had complete M1 MCA recanalization with a low-resistance waveform and improved flow velocities, also suggestive of some distal reperfusion (Figure 3.3, Frame 4). By 37 minutes, the patient could lift her arm with a mild drift, verbalize simple words, and follow axial and extra-axial commands (NIHSS score 8). However, TCD also showed multiple microembolic signals (Figure 3.3, Frame 4), suggesting continuing thrombus dissolution in the ICA and brain re-embolization from a proximal source.

At 42 minutes of infusion, TCD waveforms changed, signifying the development of re-occlusion of the M1 MCA and dampening (or suppression) of the terminal ICA flow (Figure 3.3, Frame 5). This was evident from the decrease in the mean flow velocities and increase in the resistance to flow (greater diminution of diastolic velocities compared to prior systolic/ diastolic proportions) while her BP remained stable. Two minutes later the patient rapidly became drowsy and resumed her eye deviation, global aphasia, and right hemiplegia (total NIHSS score 24).

Of note, this observation of neurological worsening during or after tPA therapy should prompt a request for urgent noncontrast head CT to rule out hemorrhagic conversion and immediate re-assessment of vitals signs for cardiac or pulmonary decompensation before TCD waveforms can be taken as evidence of re-occlusion.

At the end of tPA infusion, a terminal ICA "T"-type occlusion was present on TCD (signal deterioration similar to Figure 3.3, Frame 2). Her repeat noncontrast head CT scan showed no bleeding and no hypoattenuation, and tPA infusion was completed without interruption.

The neurological deterioration, re-occlusion process, and expected burden of atherothrombosis were explained to the family and they consented for endovascular procedures. Urgent catheter angiography showed a thrombus with an underlying atheromatous lesion in the proximal ICA and a complete terminal ICA "T"-type occlusion with no flow in the M1 MCA and A1 ACA segments (Figure 3.3, Frame 5, DSA image). Under an Institutional Review Board (IRB)-approved experimental protocol at that time, she received an additional 6 mg of intra-arterial tPA with mechanical clot disruption, leading to complete distal ICA, proximal M1 MCA, and A1 ACA recanalization with a remaining distal M1 MCA occlusion that was refractory to endovascular procedures. She also had a proximal ≥80% ICA stenosis caused by an ulcerated atheromatous plaque where the thrombus has initially formed. Diagnostic workup showed no other etiology for stroke apart from large-vessel atherothrombosis. At 2 weeks, her major deficits included aphasia and arm plegia (total NIHSS 18).

This was the first case of an arterial re-occlusion observed in real time in a stroke patient treated with fibrinolytic therapy, and it sparked the first series showing that this phenomenon could be relatively frequent with systemic thrombolytic therapy [18]. Early arterial re-occlusion was linked in real time to changes in the NIHSS scale and it is now recognized as one of the causes of early neurological deterioration or symptom fluctuation [19]. Together with persisting arterial occlusion [20] seen as failure of systemic fibrinolytics, early re-occlusion provides further arguments to pursue the development of therapies adjuvant to tPA in the lysis of thrombi and maintenance of arterial patency, as well as faster and more effective endovascular tools for reperfusion.

However, re-occlusion can occur after successful endovascular interventions [21, 22] and noninvasive repeated assessment of intracranial vessels after intravenous or endovascular treatment is advisable [17, 23]. Vascular imaging needs to be repeated if neurological deterioration or fluctuation occurs without evidence of bleeding or mass effect. Re-occlusion and persisting occlusion remain the challenge where multimodal imaging and bedside assessment skills are necessary to quickly arrive at diagnosis and mechanism, and attempt corrective measures.

Case study 3.4 Persisting arterial occlusion despite endovascular intervention

A 6-year-old boy presented to the emergency room of an outside hospital 30 minutes after the onset of left hemiparesis and dysarthria (for additional discussion, see reference [24]). He recently had mitral valve repair and ventricular septal defect closure. His father died from an ischemic stroke 2 weeks prior. Baseline NIHSS score was 15. Emergent brain CT was normal and CTA showed right TICA occlusion. The patient received i.v. tPA at a dose of 0.9 mg/kg, 10% bolus at 83 minutes after stroke onset. He did not improve by the end of tPA infusion, and therefore he was air-transferred to our center.

On arrival, his NIHSS score was 17. His mother consented for endovascular procedures and we continuously monitored his intracranial vessels with power motion Doppler TCD (PMD–TCD). Diagnostic angiography confirmed TICA occlusion (Figure 3.4). On TCD, residual TICA flow was seen as the minimal signal (systolic spikes with no diastolic flow). TCD also showed cross-filling from the left hemisphere to the right through the anterior communicating artery and detectable proximal A2 ACA flow on the right. Intra-arterial 1.1 U reteplase was given 205 minutes after symptom onset, but it did not improve flow. A Merci™ retriever was then deployed in an attempt to remove the embolus. Even after a successful pass of the device beyond the embolus (Figure 3.5) with proximal balloon inflation and aspiration the embolus was not retrieved. Over the next 60 minutes, multiple Merci™ passes were performed. Each deployment resulted in only temporary, but significant, increase in the right MCA flow velocities and appearance of positive diastolic flow. The embolus thus acted like a ball valve that could be temporarily pulled into the ICA so that flow to the MCA could be restored via the anterior cross-filling. But just like a ball valve, with any antegrade pressure it would then move back and re-occlude the MCA origin as soon as the retriever pulled through.

Because TCD was showing that the anterior communicating artery was continuously patent and provided detectable flow in the proximal A2 ACA (Figure 3.4), the decision was made to push the embolus into the proximal A1 segment to save the MCA. This was accomplished with a 3-mm Power-Sail balloon 270 min after onset. TCD provided continuous monitoring of the residual flow in the right MCA and ACA, demonstrating the advantage of multidepth simultaneous flow intensity and direction display on PMD. This information was essential to come up with the plan to "park" the embolus and to carry out this maneuver. The key to this successful repositioning of the embolus was the observation of an immediate increase in right MCA flow velocities on TCD as soon as the embolus was pushed into the right ACA. At the same time, flow in the proximal right A2 ACA continued to be uninterrupted due to the anterior cross-filling just distal to the new embolus location. A post-treatment angiogram demonstrated total recanalization of the right MCA and occlusion of the right A1 ACA (Figure 3.6).

At 24 hours his total NIHSS score was 9 points. Repeat head CT showed no hemorrhage. MRI showed an acute cortical infarction in the distribution of right MCA with no bleeding (Figure 3.6). No intracardiac thrombus was found. At 3 months, his total NIHSS score was 2 points for a left facial droop and mild sensory deficit, and he was functionally

(Continued)

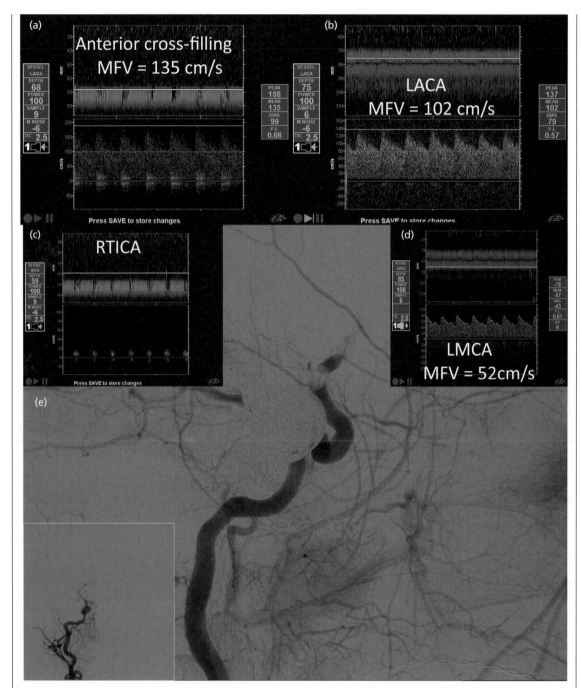

Figure 3.4 TCD and catheter angiography findings in a 6-year-old boy after completion of the intravenous tPA infusion. (a) Power motion Doppler (PMD) findings of the partial left-to-right anterior cross-filling via the anterior communicating artery (ACommA). (b) Left anterior cerebral artery (ACA) has mean flow velocity (MFV) greater than the left middle cerebral artery (MCA) (d) and pulsatility less than the MCA, findings consistent with compensatory flow increase in the donor vessel (left-to-right cross-filling). (c) PMD image shows a minimal flow signal in the right TICA, indicating persisting arterial occlusion despite receiving i.v. tPA. (e) Catheter angiographic images show the right carotid "T" occlusion.

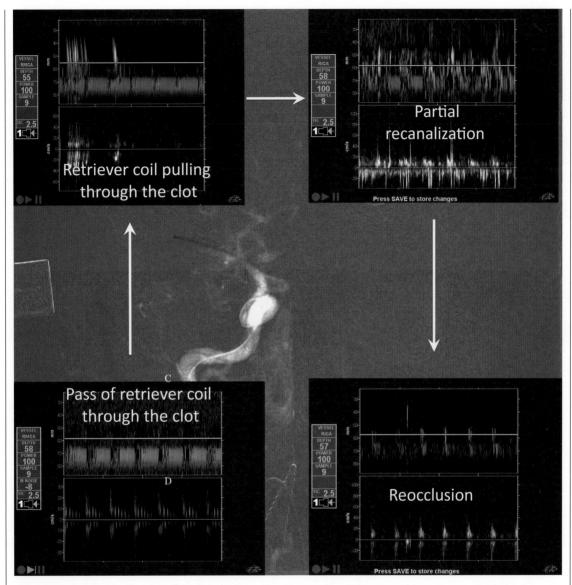

Figure 3.5 Sequential deployment of the Merci™ retriever, partial recanalization, and re-occlusion during endovascular reperfusion. TCD show sequential real time findings (arrows). Catheter angiography shows persistence of the occlusion after reperfusion attempts.

independent (modified Rankin Scale score of 1). He returned to school and has no restrictions in physical activity or learning disabilities.

This case posed the challenge of persisting arterial occlusion, for which at that time technologies like aspiration thrombectomy [25] or stentrievers [26]

were not yet available. Knowing that the anterior cross-filling from left to right was in place helped reduce the number of catheterizations of the nonaffected carotid system, and the evidence of uninterrupted flow in the right A2 ACA further helped to devise an unorthodox solution. After this case, we

(*Continued*)

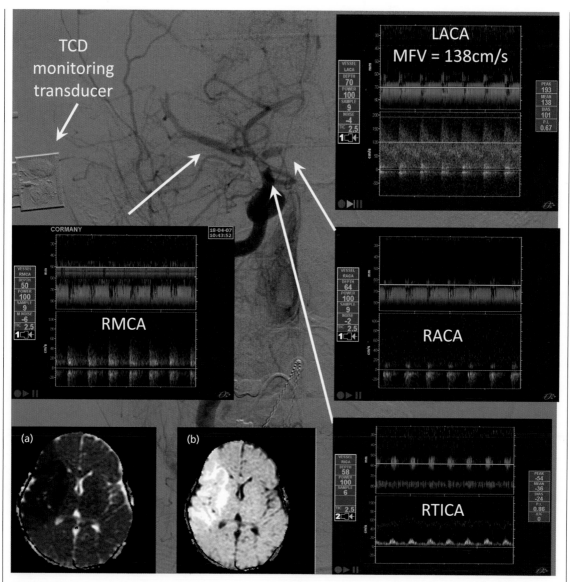

Figure 3.6 Re-positioning of the thrombus into the right A1 ACA. This maneuver was possible due to demonstration of the partial left-to-right anterior cross-filling being present and unaffected by the new thrombus location. Catheter angiography shows persisting distal A1 ACA occlusion, recanalization of the right TICA and M1 MCA. Time corresponding PMD–TCD findings are marked accordingly. (**a**, **b**) Apparent diffusion coefficient (ADC) and diffusion weighted imaging (DWI) findings after endovascular procedures.

started to monitor our endovascular interventions [17], particularly the ones that posed challenges including re-occlusion. We summarized TCD findings that could detect potentially harmful hemodynamic changes during endovascular procedures, including air embolism, re-occlusion, hyperemic reperfusion, and prolonged decreases in the residual flow due to catheter manipulations [17]. TCD surveillance shortly after endovascular procedures may also yield results that can change management.

Case study 3.5 Re-occlusion and persisting arterial occlusion after successful thrombus aspiration

A 73-year-old man developed atrial fibrillation after aortic valve replacement (for additional discussion, see reference [27]). On postoperative day 6, he developed sudden confusion, slurred speech, left facial droop, left hemiparesis, and hemineglect with a total NIHSS score of 17 points. A noncontrast head CT showed hyperdense right M1 MCA, and CT perfusion showed a large right MCA territory hypoperfusion without an established infarction (Figure 3.7). TCD found systolic spikes and absent diastolic flow at 55 mm depth in the right MCA consistent with an acute occlusion. Intravenous tPA was contraindicated due to his recent surgery and the patient was taken for mechanical thrombectomy. Diagnostic catheter angiography confirmed the right M1 MCA occlusion (Figure 3.8), and thrombus retrieval was initiated 80 minutes from stroke symptom onset. A Penumbra™ catheter was deployed once, leading to the proximal MCA recanalization and Thrombolysis in Myocardial Infarction (TIMI) grade IIb reperfusion (Figure 3.8a,b). Neurological examination 10 minutes later showed improvement to NIHSS 3 while TCD showed an improvement from the minimal flow signal with absent diastolic flow to a disturbed turbulent flow signal consistent with the residual stenosis (Figure 3.8a1,b1). The patient was given 325 mg aspirin.

Surveillance TCD monitoring was continued, and 30 minutes after completion of the thrombectomy procedure, a sudden decrease of the right MCA velocity was noted back to disappearance of the diastolic flow (Figure 3.8c1) with the patient's neurological deficit returning back to the total NIHSS score of 17 points. An angiogram confirmed re-occlusion of the right M1 MCA with some filling of the inferior division (Figure 3.8c). A Penumbra™ system was reapplied and an angiogram showed partial recanalization of the right MCA with a small thrombus within the proximal anterior temporal branch (Figure 3.8d), which is beyond the reach of the device, and the intervention was stopped. TCD continued to show delay in the systolic flow acceleration in the right M1 MCA signals with TIBI 2 flow, indicating persistence of the MCA obstruction (Figure 3.8d1). Neurologically, the patient remained unchanged. An intravenous loading dose of abciximab (20 mg) was given, followed by continuous infusion for 12 hours (0.125 μg/kg/min). TCD monitoring was continued and 1 hour later, the right MCA flow velocity increased with signs of turbulence and bruit indicating continuing recanalization (Figure 3.8e). Repeat neurological examinations started to show progressive improvement to a total NIHSS score of 3 points. At 16 hours after the second

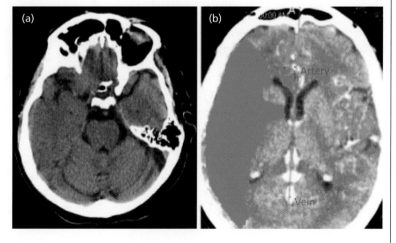

Figure 3.7 Noncontrast head CT and CT-perfusion before endovascular reperfusion procedures.
(**a**) Noncontrast CT with hyperdense right MCA sign; (**b**) large hypoperfusion defect on CT-perfusion without infarction as predicted by the commercial prognostic map software.

(Continued)

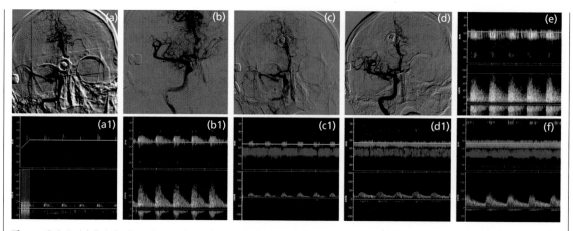

Figure 3.8 Serial digital subtraction angiography images (**a–d**) and TCD waveforms. Explanations for each image (**a–f**) are provided in the text.

intra-arterial procedure, TCD showed normal wave-form appearance in the right M1 MCA (Figure 3.8f), and the patient's total NIHSS score was 2 points (left facial droop and mild pronator drift). Repeat head CT scan showed hypodensities in the right fronto-temporal and insular territories with no hemorrhagic transformation (Figure 3.9). Subsequently, he was discharged home and his modified Rankin Scale was 1 at 6-week follow-up.

This case demonstrated that incomplete thrombus removal provides the setting for re-occlusion previously noted to occur in 15% of patients receiving endovascular procedures for acute ischemic stroke [21]. Our case further posed a challenge of persisting occlusion despite the second successful deployment of mechanical thrombectomy. Technical inability to reach the thrombus put further pressure on making a decision to go beyond the standard of care (which our patient already received when he was given 325 mg aspirin after the first procedure). TCD demonstration of persisting occlusion provided further support to initiate infusion of GPIIb–IIIa receptor antagonist. Subsequent TCD surveillance showed continuing recanalization while on abciximab, which resulted in good neurological recovery despite a large MCA infarct that matured on CT without hemorrhagic transformation. Persisting arterial occlusion and re-occlusion after endovascular procedures will remain a challenge in years to come and further adjuvant therapies should be

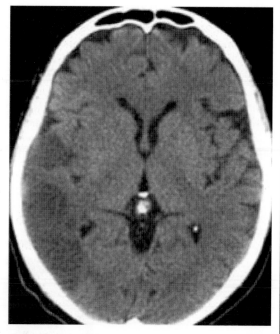

Figure 3.9 Noncontrast head CT. Infarct without hemorrhagic transformation after re-occlusion treatment with endovascular intervention and abciximab.

developed to sustain the lumen after revascularization and facilitate continuing thrombolysis in case of incomplete thrombus removal. Ultrasound offers noninvasive ways to monitor vessel patency and re-occlusion detection, and should be utilized postprocedure, particularly in intubated patients.

Case study 3.6 Recurrent aphasia with persisting proximal ICA occlusion after thrombolysis

A 56-year-old Caucasian man developed a right-sided weakness and speech arrest and was brought to our Emergency Department at 2 hours and 20 minutes from symptom onset. His head CT scan was normal, TCD showed a minimal flow signal in the left M1 MCA, and carotid duplex showed a complete ICA occlusion with pre-existing atheroma. His total NIHSS score was 22 and he received intravenous tPA at 2 hours and 53 minutes from symptom onset. Continuous TCD monitoring showed complete left MCA recanalization at 3 hours and 27 minutes with persisting proximal ICA obstruction (MCA mean flow velocity (MFV) >20 cm/s with delayed systolic flow acceleration and low resistance to flow). His NIHSS score decreased to 3 points accounting only for the right facial droop, slurred speech, and pronator drift. The head of the bed was maintained flat for 24 hours and he was admitted to the Stroke Unit.

Next morning he woke up mute. Repeat head CT showed no hemorrhage and no hypoattenuation. TCD showed sustained tenuous low-velocity blunted flow signals in the left MCA (Figure 3.10) and carotid duplex showed a complete left ICA occlusion.

Routine EEG was normal. He regained his speech in the afternoon. Next morning he was found mute again. We repeated TCD with breath holding and approximately 17 seconds into voluntary breath holding (he was able to follow commands) his MCA waveform disappeared and there was no detectable flow until he re-started breathing. This was a paradoxical reaction to increasing levels of arterial carbon dioxide. Normally, CO_2 induces arteriolar dilation and this in turn decreases resistance to flow in the proximal vessels, producing velocity increase of the incoming flow. Our patient paradoxically decreased the left MCA velocity during breath holding – this gave us an idea that his normal vessels dilated more efficiently and stole the blood flow from an artery distal to an arterial occlusion. We termed this arterial blood flow steal phenomenon leading to the neurological deterioration the "reversed Robin Hood" syndrome for analogy to "rob the poor to feed the rich" [28].

We asked his family if he stops breathing at night and they confirmed that he stops very frequently, sometimes for up to one minute. We explained that

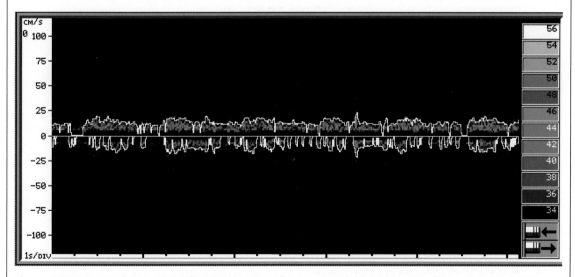

Figure 3.10 MCA waveform on TCD is flattened like venous flow or extremely blunted. This waveform was obtained distal to a carotid occlusion indicating poor ability of the circle of Willis and other collaterals to supply the MCA.

(Continued)

he likely had sleep apnea and we started him on bilevel positive airway pressure (BPAP) support at night and his aphasia did not recur. Our case illustrates the detection of a hemodynamic mechanism of neurological fluctuation in real time, and it sparked subsequent published series and led us on a quest to determine how to correct this phenomenon [29–31]. Subsequent research established this intracranial hemodynamic steal phenomenon as the missing link between sleep disordered breathing and neurological deterioration after ischemic stroke [32].

If these examples of bedside assessment and quick decision making have sparked your interest in mastering neurovascular examination with the aid of ultrasound, this book will provide you with further assistance in understanding the applied principles of ultrasound physics, hemodynamics, scanning protocols, diagnostic criteria, waveform interpretation, and differential diagnosis with discussion of the neurological and correlative neuroimaging findings. The final chapter also provides more case-based problem solving in stroke patients.

References

1. The National Institutes of Neurological Disorders and Stroke rt-PA Stroke Study Group. Tissue plasminogen activator for acute ischemic stroke. *N Engl J Med* 1995; **333**: 1581–7.

2. Hacke W, Kaste M, Fieschi C, *et al*. Intravenous thrombolysis with recombinant tissue plasminogen activator for acute hemispheric stroke. The European Cooperative Acute Stroke Study (ECASS). *JAMA* 1995; **274**: 1017–25.

3. Alexandrov AV, Demchuk A, Wein T, *et al*. The yield of transcranial Doppler in acute cerebral ischemia. *Stroke* 1999; **30**: 1605–9.

4. Caplan LR, Mohr JP, Kistler JP, *et al*. Should thrombolytic therapy be the first-line treatment for acute ischemic stroke? Thrombolysis – not a panacea for ischemic stroke. *N Engl J Med* 1997; **337**: 1309–10.

5. Demchuk AM, Felberg RA, Alexandrov AV. Clinical recovery from acute ischemic stroke after early reperfusion of the brain with intravenous thrombolysis. *N Engl J Med* 1999; **340**: 894–5.

6. Demchuk AM, Wein TH, Felberg RA, *et al*. Evolution of rapid middle cerebral artery recanalization during intravenous thrombolysis for acute ischemic stroke. *Circulation* 2000; **100**: 2282–3.

7. Burgin WS, Alexandrov AV. Deterioration following improvement with TPA therapy: carotid thrombosis and re-occlusion. *Neurology* 2001; **56**: 568–70.

8. Alexandrov AV, Molina CA, Grotta JC, *et al*. Ultrasound-enhanced systemic thrombolysis for acute ischemic stroke. *N Engl J Med* 2004; **351**: 2170–8.

9. Barreto AD, Alexandrov AV. Adjunctive and alternative approaches to current reperfusion therapy. *Stroke* 2012; **43**: 591–8.

10. Alexandrov AV, Demchuk AM, Felberg RA, *et al*. High rate of complete recanalization and dramatic clinical recovery during TPA infusion when continuously monitored by 2 MHz transcranial Doppler monitoring. *Stroke* 2000; **31**: 610–14.

11. Haley EC Jr, Lewandowski C, Tilley BC. Myths regarding the NINDS rt-PA Stroke Trial: setting the record straight. *Ann Emerg Med* 1997; **30**: 676–82.

12. Saqqur M, Tsivgoulis G, Molina CA, *et al*. for the CLOTBUST Investigators. Symptomatic intracerebral hemorrhage and recanalization after IV rt-PA: a multicenter study. *Neurology* 2008; **71**: 1304–12.

13. Ahmed N, Wahlgren N, Brainin M, *et al*. SITS Investigators. Relationship of blood pressure, antihypertensive therapy, and outcome in ischemic stroke treated with intravenous thrombolysis: retrospective analysis from Safe Implementation of Thrombolysis in Stroke–International Stroke Thrombolysis Register (SITS–ISTR). *Stroke* 2009; **40**: 2442–9.

14. Spence JD, Del Maestro RF. Hypertension in acute ischemic strokes. Treat. *Arch Neurol* 1985; **42**: 1000–2.

15. Grotta JC, Burgin WS, El-Mitwalli A, *et al*. Intravenous tissue-type plasminogen activator therapy for ischemic stroke: Houston experience 1996 to 2000. *Arch Neurol* 2001; **58**: 2009–13.

16. Tsivgoulis G, Frey JL, Flaster M, *et al*. Pre-tissue plasminogen activator blood pressure levels and risk of symptomatic intracerebral hemorrhage. *Stroke* 2009; **40**: 3631–4.

17. Rubiera M, Cava L, Tsivgoulis G, *et al*. Diagnostic criteria and yield of real time transcranial Doppler (TCD) monitoring of intra-arterial (IA) reperfusion procedures. *Stroke* 2010; **41**: 695–9.

18. Alexandrov AV, Grotta JC. Arterial re-occlusion in stroke patients treated with intravenous tissue plasminogen activator. *Neurology* 2002; **59**: 862–7.

19. Saqqur M, Molina CA, Salam A, *et al*. Clinical deterioration after intravenous recombinant tissue pasminogen activator treatment. A multicenter transcranial Doppler study. *Stroke* 2007; **38**: 69–74.

20. Smith WS, Tsao JW, Billings ME, *et al*. Prognostic significance of angiographically confirmed large vessel intracranial occlusion in patients presenting with acute brain ischemia. *Neurocrit Care* 2006; **4**: 14–17.

21. Qureshi AI, Siddiqui AM, Kim SH, *et al*. Reocclusion of recanalized arteries during intra-arterial thrombolysis for acute ischemic stroke. *AJNR Am J Neuroradiol* 2004; **25**: 322–8.

22. Qureshi AI, Hussein HM, Abdelmoula M, *et al*. Subacute recanalization and reocclusion in patients with acute ischemic stroke following endovascular treatment. *Neurocrit Care* 2009; **10**: 195–203.

23. Alexandrov AV, Sloan MA, Tegeler CH, *et al*. for the American Society of Neuroimaging Practice Guidelines Committee. Practice standards for transcranial Doppler (TCD) ultrasound. Part II. Clinical indications and expected outcomes. *J Neuroimaging* 2012; **22**: 215–24.

24. Tsivgoulis G, Horton JA, Ness JM, *et al*. Intravenous thrombolysis followed by intra-arterial thrombolysis and mechanical thrombectomy for the treatment of pediatric ischemic stroke. *J Neurol Sci* 2008; **275**: 151–3.

25. Penumbra Pivotal Stroke Trial Investigators. The penumbra pivotal stroke trial: safety and effectiveness of a new generation of mechanical devices for clot removal in intracranial large vessel occlusive disease. *Stroke* 2009; **40**: 2761–8.

26. Saver JL, Jahan R, Levy EI, *et al*. for the SWIFT Trialists. Solitaire flow restoration device versus the Merci Retriever in patients with acute ischaemic stroke (SWIFT): a randomised, parallel-group, non-inferiority trial. *Lancet* 2012; **380**: 1241–9.

27. Zhao L, Rubiera M, Harrigan MR, *et al*. Arterial re-cclusion and ersistent distal occlusion after thrombus aspiration. *J Neuroimaging* 2012; **22**: 92–4.

28. Alexandrov AV, Sharma VK, Lao AY, *et al*. Reversed Robin Hood syndrome in acute ischemic stroke patients. *Stroke* 2007; **38**: 3045–8.

29. Alexandrov AV, Ngyuen TH, Rubiera M, *et al*. Prevalence and risk factors associated with reversed Robin Hood syndrome in acute ischemic stroke. *Stroke* 2009; **40**: 2738–42.

30. Palazzo P, Balucani C, Barlinn K, *et al*. Association fo reversed Robin Hood syndrome with risk of stroke recurrence. *Neurology* 2010; **75**: 2003–8.

31. Tsivgoulis G, Zhang Y, Alexandrov AW, *et al*. Safety and tolerability of early noninvasive ventilatory correction using bilevel positive airway pressure in acute ischemic stroke. *Stroke* 2011; **42**: 1030–4.

32. Barlinn K, Alexandrov AV. Sleep-disordered breathing and arterial blood flow steal represent linked therapeutic targets in cerebral ischaemia. *Int J Stroke* 2011; **6**: 40–1

4 Applied Principles of Ultrasound Physics

"The only test I failed in my whole medical career was that on ultrasound physics."

> Frequent comment by ultrasound technology examinees

Introduction

When I was at school, I dreamed of being a physicist. My physics teacher mesmerized me by explaining how Nature works. However, it was my junior school classmate and friend, Vladimir Voevodsky, a brilliant math wizard and now at the Institute for Advanced Study in Princeton, NJ, whose extraordinary abilities across the sciences made me realize early on that physics is beyond my limits. Physics remained the area to listen, learn, absorb, and try to understand how Nature works. So humbled, I decided to become a physician. This chapter provides a simplistic introduction for clinicians to a much broader and evolving knowledge about ultrasound, a small fraction of which is used in cerebrovascular imaging.

By definition, waves are cyclic events that consist of pressure ups and downs that compress and relax the medium, supposedly leaving particles at the end of a cycle in the exact same location. Yet, when sound as a mechanical pressure wave propagates though a human body, many factors come into play and the wave eventually attenuates due to absorption and dispersion. Does the wave sent on a straight course always stay that way? Changes in direction can occur, as will be described later in this chapter. Because attenuation occurs as the wave propagates, is the energy being transformed into heat or could it interact

with tissues in other potentially harmful ways? Thermal and nonthermal bioeffects are indeed of concern and regulations apply to limit emitted ultrasound power.

For a clinician set to use ultrasound, it is important to understand the very basic principles of applied physics to explain, if need be, how a simple diagnostic ultrasound test works and why it is safe. For a scientist, examination of the human body with ultrasound offers a puzzle comparable in possibilities to a chess game or an exploration of our universe in terms of myriad of objects scattered yet interconnected across the continuum.

To begin any exploration, decide on a starting point, and where you'd like to go. If lost, always have an opportunity to come back to the starting point and rethink the strategy. This is true for skills in performance of a hand-held ultrasound test. When setting a course, have a road map (a protocol), think where you'd like to end up (assessment of target tissues and vessels), set the goal as high as possible (always generate an optimized waveform or images of the best possible quality), and perform as complete and thorough examination as possible. If going gets tough, you can settle for less but you would still end up farther from where you were at the beginning of the journey or from where you would be if you had set only a minimal goal.

However, I digress. Ultrasound has been a blessing for clinicians, and a stepchild to other imaging techniques such as CT and MRI (after triangulation and attenuation were figured out by scientists for these physical phenomena). Part of the reason for CT and MRI being easier to model and compute is that the

Neurovascular Examination: The Rapid Evaluation of Stroke Patients Using Ultrasound Waveform Interpretation, First Edition.
Andrei V. Alexandrov.
© 2013 Andrei V. Alexandrov. Published 2013 by Blackwell Publishing Ltd.

response elicited from an entire target tissue can be acquired "hands-free" using aligned emitters/ receivers of energy. We are now coming to realize that there are more ways to deliver, receive, and process ultrasound waves than was possible just a couple of decades ago. Entering the digital age, merging physics with mathematics and computing power will grant insights into the real-time functions of the human body beyond our current imagination.

Of course, the above paragraph was for the young generation, to attract more talent into the ever-growing vascular physiology and ultrasound field. And I'm not kidding!

I'm now going back to look at ultrasound wave propagation. Here are some simple facts. What is the average speed of sound in soft tissues? It is 1540 m/s, about a mile a second. What is the range of speeds? The speed is as low as 1200 m/s in cerebrospinal fluid and as high as 4400 m/s in bone such as the cranium. Obviously, there has to be a correction for this variation in arrival time of the returned echoes in order to create a high-resolution intracranial ultrasound image. Is this carried out similarly by every machine? Is there a potential for error? Always try to use the equipment yourself and get a feel for how it performs in your hands.

When learning medical ultrasound and trying to interpret an image or waveform, the best first answer you can give when results of a test are unusual or ambiguous is: "It is a technical error!" This answer implies the best and the worst in human nature. The best is that we can discover things. The worst is that these findings may not be true as they can be a product of our imagination, misunderstanding, ignorance, or blind belief. At the beginning of the learning curve I view technical errors as an opportunity to find what you did wrong and improve your knowledge and performance.

Therefore, when applying your skill, knowledge, or opinion, do the following. First, observe. Second, be open-minded. And, third, it would not hurt you to look at the literature for information or ask someone else for advice.

Basic concepts

Ultrasound is a range of frequencies above audible sound waves, that is above 20 kHz. Sound of any frequency is a mechanical wave that requires a medium in which to travel, because it squeezes and stretches the medium – that is the peak pressure compresses or rarefies matter. In other words, a single ultrasound cycle consists of the peak positive and negative pressures, as shown in Figure 4.1. The number of these cycles in a single pulse will determine the **frequency** of the emitted ultrasound beam. Ultrasound waves are termed **longitudinal** waves because particles move back and forth in the same direction as the wave.

To generate a mechanical pressure wave from an electric pulse, a piezoelectric crystal is placed in a transducer. The **piezoelectric effect** is the ability of a material to generate voltage if it is mechanically deformed, and vice versa. To transfer ultrasound energy from the transducer to soft tissues more efficiently, its surface should be coupled with skin using ultrasound transmission gel without air bubbles in it. An even interface between transducer and skin overlaying soft tissues creates better scanning conditions. A tight interface between the transcranial transducer and scalp helps to transmit more energy through the bone.

To produce an ultrasound image or spectral waveform, the wave needs a reflector. If the reflector is weak (like red blood cells in Figure 4.1, schematically depicted under "Reflection"), the echo is weak and the object may not be detected. Note that moving red blood cells appear dark on brightness-modulated (**B-mode**) images because the amplitude of the reflected echoes is much weaker than those originating from

Transducer Pressure Pulse Wave Propagation Reflection Absorption

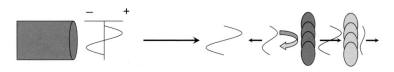

Figure 4.1 Longitudinal ultrasound wave travel in soft tissues.

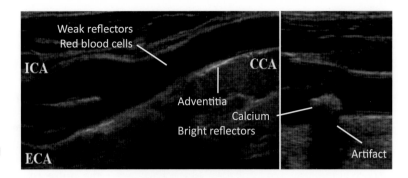

Figure 4.2 B-mode imaging of carotid bifurcations and strength of tissue reflectors. CCA, common carotid artery; ECA, external carotid artery; ICA, internal carotid artery.

vessel walls (Figure 4.2). If the reflector is too strong or "bright", that is calcium, an artifact such as **shadowing** can occur (Figure 4.2, right image). This means that the reflector destroyed antegrade wave propagation and practically no echoes can be detected beyond the reflector.

Ultrasound waves are describes through **acoustic parameters** (Box 4.1). Period and frequency are determined by the sound source only; amplitude, power, and intensity are initially determined by the source but as the wave propagates through soft tissues, it attenuates and these parameters decrease (so the medium absorbs or dissipates energy carried by a ultrasound wave); wavelength is the only parameter that is determined by both the source and the medium; and propagation speed is determined by the medium.

Propagation speed is determined by **stiffness** and **density** of the medium. Stiffer objects resist compression better than soft objects and ultrasound travels faster. Propagation speed is directly proportional to stiffness. However, as density increases, objects become heavier and sound waves slow down. Propagation speed is inversely proportionate to density. In general, sound waves travel faster in solids, then liquids, then gases.

The higher the ultrasound frequency, the shorter the wavelength because more cycles have to be packed in a pulse. The shorter the wavelength, the greater the attenuation because the wave encounters more objects in soft tissues comparable to the wavelength in size. The lower the frequency, the lower the resolution of an image. Yet lower frequencies, such as 1–2 MHz, offer better Doppler velocity sampling and emboli detection compared to the higher frequencies that are more commonly used for color flow or structural grayscale imaging in vascular ultrasound. Also, lower fre-

---

Box 4.1 Definitions of the acoustic parameters

Period: Time that it takes a wave to vibrate in a single cycle (single pulse duration), or the time from the start of a cycle to the start of the next cycle (pulse repetition period); measured in microseconds for medical diagnostic ultrasound.

Frequency: The number of cycles that occur in 1 second; measured in Hertz (1 cycle / 1 second = 1 Hertz); range kHz (therapeutic) and MHz (therapeutic and diagnostic ultrasound).

Amplitude: The difference between the maximum positive or negative values over the undisturbed value for pressure (measured in Pascals), density (measured in g/cm^3), or particle motion or distance (measured in mm or cm).

Power: The rate of energy transfer, i.e. rate at which work is performed; measured in Watts; range under 700 mW for diagnostic ultrasound.

Intensity: The concentration of energy in the sound beam, i.e. power distribution in the area the beam is applied to; measured in W/cm^2.

Wavelength: The spatial length of a single complete pulse cycle; inversely related to frequency; measured in mm or cm.

Propagation speed: The distance that ultrasound travels in 1 second; measured in m/s; average speed of ultrasound in soft tissues is 1540 m/s or "a mile a second".

---

quencies offer better penetration through the skull bone, thus making brain imaging possible with echocardiographic transducers (2–4 MHz). Because lower frequencies penetrate better, they are also used to image deeper structures in the body compared to higher frequencies.

Pressure

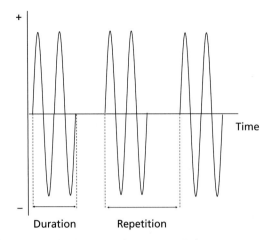

Time

Duration   Repetition

Figure 4.3 Pulse duration and repetition periods.

Before embarking on factors that affect resolution of ultrasound images, a fundamental concept of pulse duration and repetition has to be discussed. Pulse itself is a collection of cycles that travel together (Figure 4.3). Pulse duration is inversely proportionate to sound frequency because it determines the number of cycles per pulse. The higher the frequency the more cycles are packed in one pulse. Typical pulse duration in diagnostic ultrasound is 2.0 microseconds or less, and sonographers cannot change this setup. However, the **pulse repetition frequency** (**PRF** = 1/ pulse repetition period) can be adjusted during examination and it is limited by imaging depth. Figure 4.4 illustrates adjustments in PRF with changes in imaging depth.

Ultrasound pulses have spatial dimensions that are determined by the footprint of the transducer and by

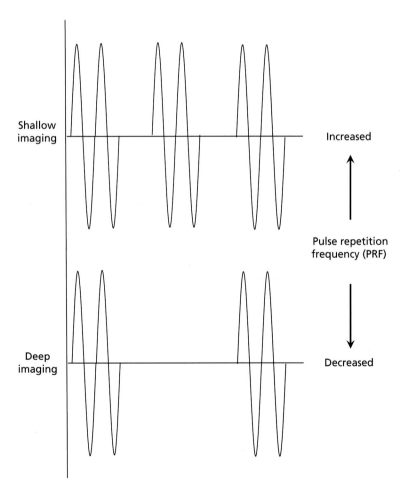

Shallow imaging

Increased

Pulse repetition frequency (PRF)

Deep imaging

Decreased

Figure 4.4 Imaging depth and pulse repetition frequency.

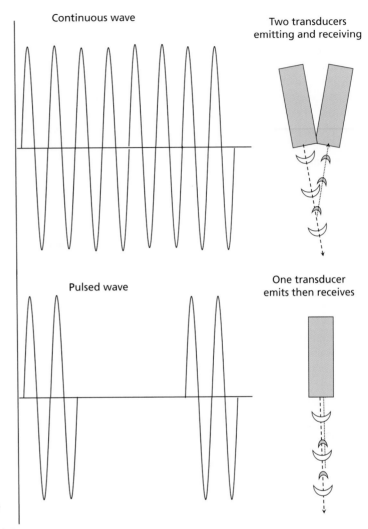

Figure 4.5 Continuous (CW) and pulsed wave (PW) ultrasound modes.

spatial pulse length, that is the distance that a pulse occupies in space from the start to the end of the pulse.

Spatial pulse length (mm) = number of cycles
$$\times \text{ wavelength (mm)}$$

Shorter pulses produce more accurate images because resolution is improved by sampling smaller amounts of tissue at a time.

To create an image or a waveform, ultrasound machine needs to send a pulse and then stop and listen to arriving echoes. This is the principle behind **pulsed wave** (PW) ultrasound. If the machine emits pulses all the time, it produces **continuous wave** (CW) ultrasound that is not good for imaging because no depth information can be derived. The percentage of time that the sound source uses to emit pulses as opposed to the listening part of the pulse repetition period is described by the **duty factor**:

Duty factor (%) = (pulse duration/
$$\text{pulse repetition period}) \times 100$$

For the continuous wave ultrasound it is 100% (Figure 4.5). Note that two transducers are required with the CW mode: one for constantly emitting sound and another for constantly receiving echoes. No depth discrimination is possible and CW is not used for imaging. PW requires only one transducer, which first emits and then detects returned echoes. Timing of the returned echoes is then used for depth discrimination.

Typically, with pulsed wave ultrasound imaging, the duty factor is 0.2–0.5%, meaning that over 99% of the time the ultrasound machine is listening as opposed to emitting pulses. However, it emits short-duration pulses thousands of times each second and that creates an illusion of real-time imaging and a constant emission of pulses. In summary, by adjusting the imaging depth or Doppler velocity scale, sonographers change the pulse repetition period, PRF, and duty factor.

How does an ultrasound machine determine the depth from which the returned echoes originated? As shown in Figure 4.6, a single-gate spectral Doppler system is able to display the depth of insonation. Several assumptions are built into sampling the returned echoes from the depth set on the spectral Doppler machine display (Figure 4.6a). First, a pulse is emitted and then the transducer becomes inactive for the time necessary for the wave to reach 64 mm depth and then for the return echoes to come back. The theoretical time for this round trip would be: distance (0.0064 m) divided by the average speed of sound in soft tissues (1540 m/s) times two for the round trip = 8.3 microseconds (Figure 4.6b). There-fore, a transcranial Doppler (TCD) unit opens the gate right about that time to listen to returned echoes. The **gate** is the time interval at which the transducer is switched to the listening mode and arriving echoes are detected, amplified, and processed. When the gate closes, the next pulse is emitted and the process is repeated many times a second (Figure 4.6c). If the listening time interval is set too short, it creates a small gate or sample volume. This can make sampling more precise (and generate sharper images with ultrasound imaging tests); however, it will limit the sensitivity of TCD to detect flow because intracranial arteries are small and any transducer movement may dislodge the beam off the intercept.

Furthermore, an ultrasound beam has three dimensions, ultrasound pulses have spatial length, and the beam encounters structures that can change propagation speed by thousands of meters per second. This creates some uncertainty and potential for error. Figure 4.7 illustrates the principle of **sample volume** or gate.

As a 2-MHz ultrasound wave leaves the transducer and goes through the **near field**, it then narrows to the beam minimal diameter in the **focal zone**. The distance from the transducer to this focus (or minimal diameter) is also known as the focal length. After a depth of 50 mm, a 2-MHz beam diverges into the far field. The beginning of beam widening marks the beginning of the **far zone** or **Fraunhofer zone**.

If the depth of insonation is also set at 50 mm, 90% of the returned Doppler signal will originate from within the 3 mm core (the black oval area depicted in Figure 4.7) and another 10% of the signal will come from the three-dimensional sample of tissues around it. Think of this **sample volume** (or **gate**) as the depth range that can be sampled. The sum of standard deviations from the set depth of insonation is the length of the sample volume along the ultrasound beam axis, that is depth 50 mm ± 5 mm yields a gate of 10 mm. This means that if a signal is detected at a depth of 50 mm it can in theory originate anywhere from within 45 mm to 55 mm depth. Obviously, the core should yield the best returned signals but a bright reflector on the periphery of the sample volume can also produce detectable echoes.

By analogy, think about an ultrasound beam like a flashlight. If you walk at night and point the flashlight at the ground, you only see the surface illuminated by the beam footprint. You can control how much you see by reducing the size of the light spot or making it larger. Although this example is more pertinent to beam focusing using a lens (which will be discussed below), changing the gate or sample volume during ultrasound exposure also changes the amount of tissues being sampled.

After echoes are detected by a single element TCD transducer, several things happen during postprocessing of the received echoes. Timing is everything. If the instrument is set to listen to only one depth of insonation, TCD provides a single-gate measurement (Figure 4.8a). Once a pulse is emitted, a TCD instrument can listen to several time epochs, and measurements will be **multigated**. Often these spectral Doppler multi-gate measurements overlap substantially (as shown in the multigate example in Figure 4.8b) where the sonographer can control and change an overlap between gates. Finally, numerous gates can be set for sampling (power motion mode TCD machines usually offer 33 to 250 gates), and flow direction as well as

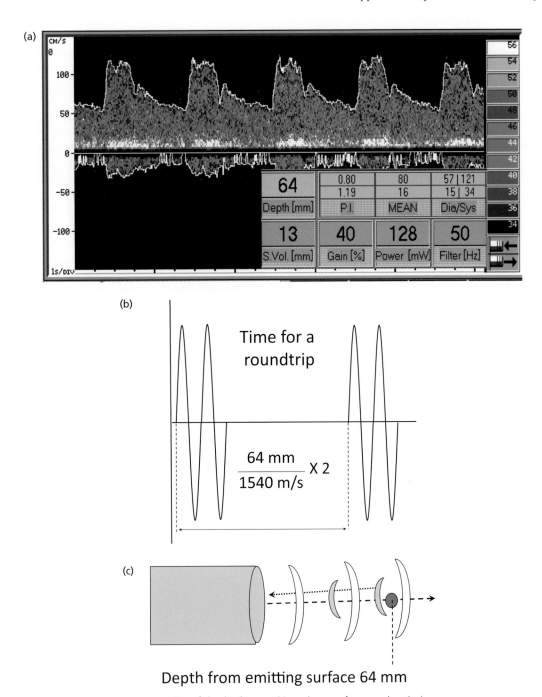

Figure 4.6 Single-gate pulsed wave sampling of the depth set at 64 mm (see text for an explanation).

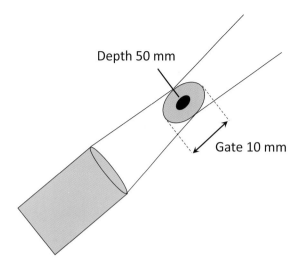

Figure 4.7. Sample volume and depth of insontaion with a single-gate TCD beam.

intensity information can be displayed (Figure 4.8c). This approach is complimentary to spectral waveform sampling and can yield additional information, which will be discussed in other chapters.

In Figure 4.8a, a single-gate TCD spectral waveform was obtained at a depth of 50 mm with 11.8 mm sample volume (Multigon Industries). Multigate spectral Doppler tracings were obtained with Companion III software (Nicolet Biomedical). Spectral windows on the left of the bottom image demonstrate waveforms at sequentially increasing depths corresponding to motion mode window displays 1A through 1H. Note the 50% overlap between adjacent gates. This affects resolution of the m-mode display. For comparison, look at the **power motion Doppler** (PMD, Spencer Technologies) image on the right. PMD utilizes 33 partially overlapping but much smaller gates that offer better resolution. Apart from flow direction, the display also includes information about the returned echoes intensity over 65 mm of intracranial space. The utility of this information for window finding and emboli tracking, as well as other applications, will be discussed in subsequent chapters. Examples in Figure 4.8 illustrate "nonimaging" TCD insonation results with a 2-MHz beam.

One can also use pulsed wave ultrasound to create structural and functional real-time images. To achieve sharp resolution, an obvious first step would be to use a small transducer footprint and deploy a higher carrying frequency, which, remember, has a shorter wavelength and can discriminate smaller reflectors. Figure 4.9 shows how a linear array of small pulsed wave transducers can be aligned to produce real-time images.

Higher frequencies are deployed for color flow imaging (range 2–3.5 MHz for transcranial imaging, 4–7 MHz for carotid flow imaging) and 4–12 MHz for gray-scale structural vascular imaging. Dark dots indicate small sample volumes or gates deployed with this form of imaging. Transducers are activated sequentially, being linearly aligned in two rows, and the emitted beams are steered electronically. Multigate sampling is deployed to detect the returned echoes.

Using gray-scale (or structural) imaging, one depicts the strength or amplitude of the returned echoes with frequency similar to the one that was emitted. This form of imaging is called brightness modulated, or **B-mode** (Figure 4.2). The accuracy of any ultrasound imaging is described as resolution. **Axial resolution** refers to the ability of a system to display two structures that are close together along (or in parallel) to the ultrasound beam axis. Axial resolution is therefore measured as the minimal distance between two objects that can produce two distinct echoes that a system can display without an artifact. Axial resolution is determined by pulse spatial length whereby shorter pulses improve axial resolution. Both the source (i.e. ultrasound transducer/ machine) and the medium (i.e. tissues through which the beam propagates) influence axial resolution (AR):

$$AR = \text{spatial pulse length (mm)}/2$$
$$= \text{wavelength (mm)} \times \text{number of cycles in a pulse}/2$$

Transducers with fewer cycles per pulse produce less "ringing" and this is achieved through dampening of the piezoelectric crystal after it is excited by the electrical signal to produce a pulse.

Another aspect of imaging accuracy is described by **lateral resolution**. Lateral resolution is the minimal distance between two objects perpendicular to the beam axis that can produce two distinct echoes that a system can display without an artifact. Lateral resolution is determined by the width of an ultrasound beam. Because the beam diameter varies with depth, lateral resolution also changes with depth. It is better

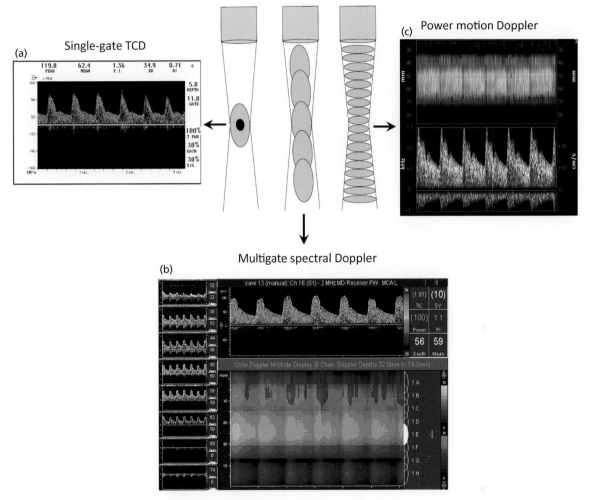

Figure 4.8 (**a**) Single and (**b, c**) multiple-gate sampling along a single ultrasound beam axis.

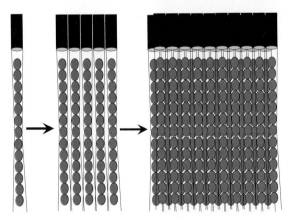

Figure 4.9 Linear array of double layer pulsed wave transducers for duplex scanning.

in the near field, best at the focal zone, and worst in the far field where the beam diverges.

Two main factors determine beam width and divergence: transducer diameter and emitted frequency. Piezoelectric crystal diameter and beam divergence are inversely related. The larger the footprint of the transducer the less the beam divergence in the far field. Lower-frequency transducers produce beams that diverge more. Higher-frequency transducers produce beams that diverge less, thus enabling duplex probes to align more crystals and generate images with better lateral resolution. However, higher frequencies also have deeper focal zones where resolution is best, while most cerebrovascular imaging is done at shallow depths of extracranial carotid vasculature. To achieve

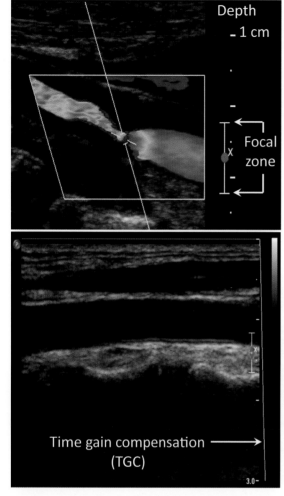

Figure 4.10 Focal zone placement with imaging of a hypoechoic plaque and residual lumen in the common carotid artery.

pronounced curvatures of the lens or crystal narrow the beam, leading to a fixed and better focusing. Phased array focusing is applied for array transducers used for duplex imaging. With the latter, sonographers can control where to place additional focal zones (Figure 4.10). Remember that a phased array produces adjustable, multifocus images.

B-mode images of the carotid arteries are rectangular because they are produced with a linear sequential array transducer. Color flow or power mode boxes can be rectangular or parallelograms (Figures 4.10 and 4.11). Transcranial duplex (or echocardiographic) transducers have a square footprint but produce sector-like images. The latter are produced with vector array transducers (Figure 4.11). These transducers combine linear sequential and linear phased array technologies to electronically steer ultrasound beams outside the footprint of the transducer. Furthermore, electronic steering can be applied to linear sequential array transducers to produce parallelogram-shaped images (Figure 4.11b). Beam formers send electric pulses to the crystals in the sequences (or slopes of the electrical pulse lines) shown in Figure 4.11a. The beam is steered if the electrical pulse spike line has a slope.

Remember, any two-dimensional image generated from a three-dimensional beam flattens or compresses structures that in reality may not be on the same plane in the body. The ultrasound beam is not razor sharp and transducers, though small, are arranged in arrays that have considerable sizes. This is governed by the **slice thickness resolution**, or elevational resolution. In other words, do objects seen on the image reside in the imaging plane or above and below it? This is also known in CT and MR imaging as the partial volume averaging artifact, which is unavoidable when one compresses adjacent projections into one two-dimensional image. With duplex imaging, this leads to over-position of blood flow signals over the plaque or vessel wall shine-through in the middle of the patent artery with off-center positioning of the ultrasound beam instead over the common carotid artery.

In the duplex image shown in Figure 4.12, blood flow signals are superimposed into plaque structure when in reality this is blood flow above a mild plaque. Furthermore, the vessel wall appearance in the middle of the vessel is likely due to the object intercepted below and also projecting into the scanning plane.

better scanning conditions for shallow structures using higher frequencies, duplex transducers are packed with very-small-diameter crystals, which produce less-deep focal zones.

To further shape up the ultrasound beam specific to the task, the following three types of **focusing** are used: external, internal, and phased array. External and internal focusing can be used with single-element transducers. External focusing is achieved by placement of a lens between the piezoelectric crystal and transducer surface. Internal focusing is accomplished by changing the curvature of the crystal itself. More-

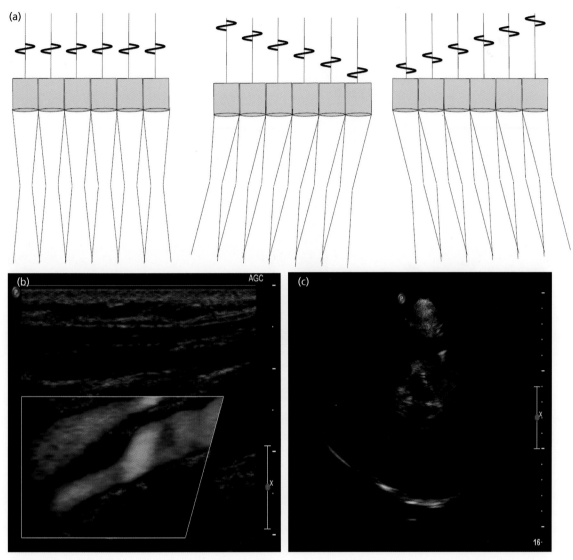

Figure 4.11 Electronic steering of ultrasound beams in cerebrovascular imaging. (**a**) Electric pulses show timing of transducer excitation. (**b**) Parallelogram power mode box depicting flow in the internal carotid artery. (**c**) Transcranial duplex image generated by an echocardiographic transducer showing butterfly-shaped brainstem and contralateral skull.

These artifacts are induced by near-wall or off-center positioning of an ultrasound beam instead of perpendicular interception of the common carotid artery through the middle of the vessel. To avoid these artifacts, remember the scanning rule: "keep both ends of the pipe open." This will be discussed further.

Artifacts represent errors in imaging that result from the physics of ultrasound, often combined with operator errors, problems with equipment, or deviations in tissue behavior from models that are used to generate images. The most common artifact seen with carotid imaging is **shadowing**, as shown in Figure 4.2. It implies that ultrasound either met a bright reflector that bounced back the wave or it simply could not pass through a structure (most often calcium or air, respectively). If located within the plaque, it

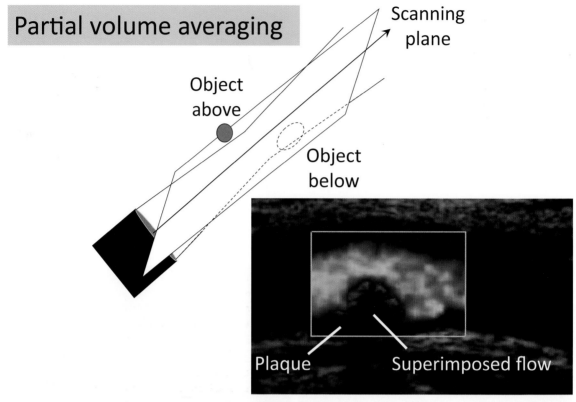

Figure 4.12 Slice thickness resolution and artifacts from reflectors above and below the scanning plane.

indicates the presence of calcium. Shadowing is also used to find transverse processes and locate the vertebral artery on the neck (Figure 4.13a). This artifact (Figure 4.13b) is also known as **edge shadow** or **shadow by refraction**. Besides refraction, beam redirection can also be caused by **Rayleigh scattering**. Both phenomena are shown below (Figure 4.14). Adventitia, intima, and adjacent red blood cells (small reflectors in the transverse projection, Figure 4.13) are responsible for expanding shadows distal to the point of ultrasound beam diversion and partial destruction. Note that these shadows originate from the outer parts of the common carotid artery transverse view where the intercepted adventitia has the smallest diameter comparable to ultrasound beam dimensions.

Refraction, or the change in the direction of ultrasound wave propagation, occurs when an ultrasound beam travels from one medium to another at certain conditions. First, the incidence angle of the beam intercepting the boundary must be oblique (Figure 4.14), and propagation speeds of the two media must be different. As a result, change in the transmission speed will cause ultrasound to travel in a different direction.

With oblique interception of a boundary between two tissues (medium 1 and 2), further direction of the beam is dependent on propagation speed difference. If speed 1 is greater than 2, the transmission angle (arrow in the green medium) is less than the incidence angle (arrow in the blue medium). If speed 1 is less than 2, the transmission angle is greater than the incidence angle. The latter is particularly true with TCD insonation through the temporal bone. If an ultrasound beam encounters an object that is comparable in its dimensions to the beam or wavelength, scattering of attenuated echoes may occur in every direction. This phenomenon is known as Rayleigh scattering, and is proportionate to the forth power of the emitted frequency. This scattering is organized and red blood cells redirect ultrasound energy in every

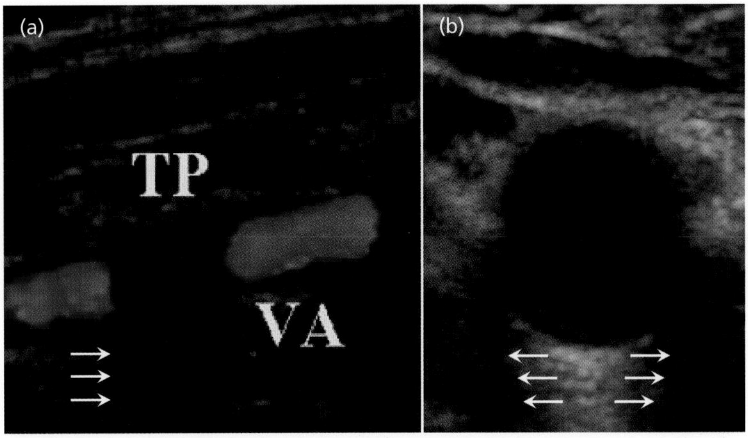

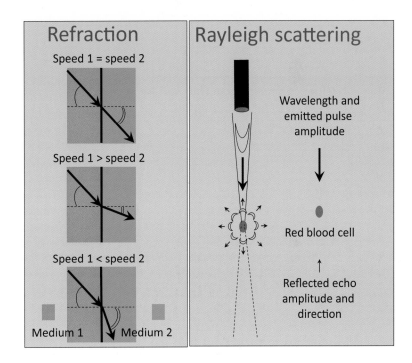

Figure 4.13 Examples of shadowing artifact with carotid and vertebral duplex scanning. (**a**) A transverse process (TP) casts a shadow over the vertebral artery (VA), and this shadow is used to locate intratransverse views of the VA. (**b**) Shadow produced by a noncalcified carotid vessel wall intercepted cross-sectionally.

Figure 4.14 Beam redirection with refraction and Rayleigh scattering.

direction. Although these phenomena are totally different, they produce changes in sound propagation and beam direction.

Refraction redirects the ultrasound beam and degrades lateral resolution. It can also produce a **refraction artifact** where a false image of a structure resides *side by side* (or at the same depth) as the real image (Figure 4.15). Ultrasound reflection and redi-

rection off a strong reflector produces an artifact known as **mirror image**. Remember that the artifact is placed *deeper* than the real structure (Figure 4.15). The real structure may not cause an artifact because another reflector, termed the mirror, is likely responsible for it. For example, reflections from pleura can produce an image of two sublavian arteries. Adventitia of the CCA can produce artificial color flow projection.

Refraction artifact

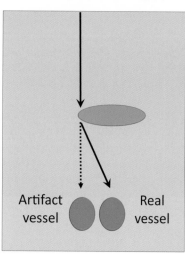

Artifact
vessel Real
vessel

Mirror artifact

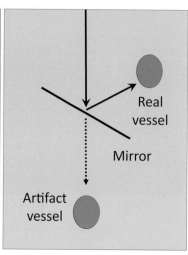

Real
vessel

Mirror

Artifact
vessel

Figure 4.15 Artifacts due to beam redirection. Green oval is a tissue with propagation speed different from surrounding structures. Mirror is a bright reflector on the beam path.

Box 4.2 Other main artifacts that can be seen with vascular duplex imaging

Reverberation: Ultrasound wave bounces between two strong reflectors producing multiple equally spaced echoes.

Comet tail: Also known as ring down artifact, it is produced by reverberation leaving solid hyperechoic lines distal to bright reflectors.

Enhancement: A structure with abnormally low attenuation produces a hyperechoic region distal to it.

Focal enhancement: Also known as focal banding artifact, it is usually seen across the image in focal zones where enhancement is greater.

Speed error: Also known as range ambiguity artifact, it is produced by ultrasound wave propagation at speeds different from 1540 m/s. As a result, structural images can be split or cut as if tissue is displaced.

Lobes: An artifact appears side-by-side with the true reflector due to sound energy transmission outside of the beam main axis.

To spot an artifact, know normal anatomy and check if suspicious sister-like images are at equal distances from the potential mirror.

Several other artifacts that can be seen with duplex imaging are summarized in Box 4.2, although the list is by no means complete. Refer to specialized text-books on ultrasound imaging physics for a complete description and further details. Doppler assessment of arterial blood flow and related artifacts will be discussed in the next chapter.

Bioeffects

The diagnostic ultrasound wave delivers a small but measurable mechanical **radiation force** to any tissue it strikes. If the ultrasound beam is absorbed or reflected, a mechanical momentum is transmitted from the wave to the tissue. This interaction between ultrasound and tissue results in a bioeffect through energy transmission. Beam intensity is most relevant to production of bioeffects, namely spatial peak temporal average (**SPTA**) intensity, which should be kept at <700 mW/cm^2 for diagnostic ultrasound. Bioeffects can be negative, that is leading to tissue damage, and therefore diagnostic ultrasound has been regulated to minimize patient risk through this intensity threshold. Bioeffects can also be positive if ultrasound helps to improve tissue healing or amplifies action of medications in a safe manner.

The two most important mechanisms that lead to bioeffects are **heating** and **cavitation**. As the ultrasound wave propagates through the body, part of the energy is absorbed through conversion into heat, that is the thermal mechanism. The **thermal index** predicts the maximum temperature raise under given insonation conditions. It is reported for the following tissues: TIS, for soft tissues; TIB, for bones; and TIC, for cranial bone. The latter could be shown on a TCD display. Diagnostic ultrasound can cause temperature elevations, usually not exceeding 2 degrees Celsius and prolonged (up to 50 hours) exposure to diagnostic ultrasound showed no damage to insonated tissues.

Cavitation describes creation of gaseous nuclei from dissolved gases in a fluid exposed to ultrasound, that is the nonthermal mechanism. Cavitation can be induced as stable or transient. Stable cavitation occurs at lower peak negative pressures when formed gaseous nuclei tend to oscillate in size but do not burst. Transient cavitation is produced by higher peak negative pressures and leads to bursting of gaseous nuclei. It is also known as inertial cavitation. The likelihood of harmful bioeffects due to cavitation is predicted by the **mechanical index** (MI). MI is related to peak negative pressure and emitted ultrasound frequency. Higher MI values are associated with greater peak negative pressures and lower frequencies. An easier way to remember what MI and TI reflect is the expression: "shake and bake" referring to cavitation and thermal effects respectively.

The American Institute of Ultrasound in Medicine (AIUM) has stated that no harmful bioeffects have been reported to date from exposure to diagnostic ultrasound. To minimize patient exposure to ultrasound energy, sonographers should follow the ALARA principle: as low as reasonably achievable. With TCD examination, this is done by reducing power of the emitted signal to 10% when investigating through the orbit, burr hole, craniotomy site, or fontanelle. A transtemporal examination through intact skull should start with 100% power, seemingly violating the ALARA principle. However, this allows a window to be found faster or to be found in a patient who has suboptimal windows, and thus the examination can be completed faster. Therefore, it satisfies the second safety precaution for diagnostic ultrasound: minimize the time of overall patient exposure to ultrasound. Furthermore, special clinical situations require continuous TCD monitoring that is safe in patients undergoing emboli detection or even receiving thrombolysis with intravenous tissue plasminogen activator. There is a possibility that even low-power diagnostic ultrasound could produce other bioeffects, such as reversible disaggregation of fibrin strands in the thrombus, increase in streaming of plasma around and through the thrombus, delivery of medications to tissues with compromised perfusion, and release of nitric oxide inducing vasodilation. Examples of harvesting both harmful and positive bioeffects include the development of high-intensity focused ultrasound (HIFU) therapeutic systems for tissue ablation through thermal and cavitational mechanisms, and sonothrombolysis for acute stroke likely through an increased tissue plasminogen activator (tPA) delivery to the thrombus, promotion of its fibrinolytic activity, and possibly vasodilation.

This brief introduction by no means covers the vast field of ultrasound physics nor all the terminology, definitions, and explanations that clinicians should know in order to perform and interpret ultrasound tests. More information can be found in specific textbooks dealing with ultrasound physics and instrumentation in the Recommended Reading list.

Recommended reading

Edelman SK. *Understanding Ultrasound Physics*, 4th edn. ESP Inc, 2012.

Kremkau F. *Sonography Principles and Instruments*, 8th edn. St Louie, Missouri: Saunders, 2010.

Valdueza JM, Shreiber SJ, Roehl JE, Klingebiel R. *Neurosonology and Neuroimaging of Stroke*. Stuttgart, Germany: Thieme, 2008.

Current study materials offered by Davies Publishing: http://www.daviespublishing.com.

5 Applied Principles of Hemodynamics

"Go with the flow."

One of ten (or more) sonographer
"shalt" commandments

Hemodynamics describes the flow of blood through the circulatory system. Blood flows from the heart through arteries to the vessels of microcirculation and returns through veins back to the heart. This is possible due to pressure gradients. Heart muscle contracts and ejects blood with a velocity that is a reflection of the kinetic pressure transmitted from the heart to accelerate blood, and with blood pressure, a form of potential energy. An additional amount of potential energy is stored through blood's gravitational properties, while moving blood also has kinetic energy. If a pool of blood is injected into a rigid system, the heart will need to work twice as hard. As we discuss the pressure–flow relationships in the circulatory system, keep in mind the properties the recipient vessel wall needs to have in order to maintain circulation and reduce the effort required of the heart, thereby to preserving the muscle to continue pumping for an entire lifetime.

In simple terms, movement of blood is analogous with an electric current. **Ohm's law** can be applied to describe flow through the vascular system. It states that blood flow is directly proportional to the pressure difference (Δ), but inversely proportional to the resistance:

Blood flow = Δ pressure/resistance

Flow of blood through a vessel is mainly determined by two factors: (1) differences in pressure ($P_1 - P_2$) between the beginning and the end of a vessel; and (2) resistance to flow.

Resistance, or impediment to flow, is affected by many factors and cannot be measured directly. It is inferred from measurements of blood flow and pressure difference within a vessel, or from the shape of the spectral waveform, which will be discussed later. Briefly, resistance can be inferred from the difference between peak systolic and end diastolic pressures or velocities, where a marked decrease in diastolic pressures signifies a rise in resistance. Resistance differs throughout the body as it is a product of changing vessel diameter, cross-sectional area, length (when affected by plaques or re-directed via collaterals), and blood viscosity. Blood **viscosity** is primarily determined by hematocrit, or the percentage of red blood cells in blood. Higher hematocrit and smaller caliber of the vessel raise resistance and impede flow, requiring higher pressures to overcome these obstacles.

As blood moves through the body, loss of energy occurs. Energy is lost through viscosity, friction, and inertial loss. The latter occurs every time the blood velocity changes. Among its many functions, endothelial lining helps reduce friction loss due to blood cells rubbing against the vessel walls. Elasticity of vessels preserves energy introduced to the system by the heart and promotes flow through the **Windkessel effect**. This effect describes the arterial system's ability to receive pulsatile energy from the heart during systolic ejection and convert this to continuous pulsating waves, which foster movement of blood through the systemic circulation. Arterial wall distensibility is the main factor responsible for maintaining the Windkessel effect on pulsatile transmission. Distensibility and the subsequent elastic recoil of arterial vessels assists constant forward flow during the diastolic phase of the cardiac cycle. This in turn reduces the

Neurovascular Examination: The Rapid Evaluation of Stroke Patients Using Ultrasound Waveform Interpretation, First Edition.
Andrei V. Alexandrov.
© 2013 Andrei V. Alexandrov. Published 2013 by Blackwell Publishing Ltd.

Parabolic

Plug-like

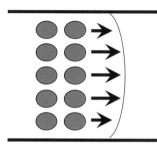

Figure 5.1 Types of laminar flow. The layer closest to the vessel wall moves at the slowest velocity. Larger vessels like the aorta or flow through a poststenotic dilation may have a plug-like flow.

Stenosis

Bifurcation

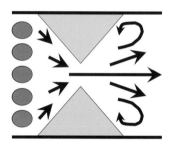
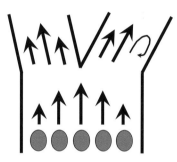

Figure 5.2 Turbulent flow in an artery. Turbulence indicates energy loss and can be found after an arterial stenosis, over a rough surface, or a sharp change in the direction of flow at bifurcations.

systemic vascular resistance (SVR) and the workload of the heart during systole. As elasticity is reduced by atherosclerosis or chronic hypertension, resistance to the arterial blood flow increases, further prompting the need for a greater wall tension and an increase in the left ventricle's workload.

The amount of muscle tension within the vascular bed necessary to maintain specific flow pressures varies significantly. According to the **law of Laplace**, the muscle tension (T) needed to maintain a specific pressure (P) is reduced if the radius (R) decreases:

$$P = T/R$$

The larger the blood vessel diameter, the more tension is required to maintain a given pressure within the vessel, that is tension in the aorta is approximately 10,000 times that within a capillary bed. This influences composition of the vessel wall and appearance of smooth muscle cells in branching arteries of smaller caliber and arterioles.

Changes in vessel diameter alter resistance and affect the movement of blood flow, leading to a phenomenon known as laminar flow or streamlining of blood velocity profile. **Laminar flow** is the parabolic or plug-like movement of blood in layers within a blood vessel (Figure 5.1).

Turbulent flow occurs when blood starts to form eddy currents, and a cross-wise as well as streamlined flow can be found (Figure 5.2).

The appearance of turbulence at a certain velocity threshold is determined by the **Reynolds number** (Re):

$$Re = 2rv\rho/\eta$$

where r is the radius of the lumen, ρ is the density of blood, and η is the fluid viscosity The higher the Reynolds number (i.e. $\geq$2000–2200 in a vessel with smooth walls) for a given velocity v, the higher the propensity to turbulence. This propensity increases with higher density of blood and lower blood viscosity. More turbulence flattens the velocity profile. Remember, turbulence increases friction and resistance.

Because turbulence produces chaotic blood currents, it cannot be quantified with current ultrasound measurements, though an experienced sonographer will immediately say that turbulence is present in a vessel by hearing a disturbed audio signal or by looking at spectral waveforms (examples could be found in subsequent chapters). Furthermore, turbulence accounts for energy losses and thus it disrupts the relationship between pressure and flow as described by Hagen–Poiseuille law and further affects the correlation between the degree of stenosis and velocity.

Hagen–Poiseuille's law describes the impact of resistance on blood flow:

$$\text{Flow rate}\ (Q) = \frac{\pi(P_1 - P_2)r^4}{8\eta L}$$

where the blood flow (Q) is directly proportional to the pressure difference across the vessel ($P_1 - P_2$), to the fourth power of the vessel radius (r^4), and is inversely proportional to the vessel length (L) and blood viscosity (η), while the $\pi/8$ ratio reflects the dependence of flow on the vessel area and circumference.

It is important to remember that a long arterial segment with a small diameter will decrease flow more effectively than a short stenosis of the same residual diameter. As an example, hypoplastic vessels carry little flow to the brain.

The heart ejects blood into the circulation through sequential electrical and mechanical events within a single heart beat, or cardiac cycle. When the heart ejects blood in systoli, arterial pressure increases, vessel walls distend, and the systemic vascular resistance decreases, leading to an increase in blood flow. A drop in arterial pressure after closure of the aortic valve induces a decrease in vessel diameter, resulting from reduced arterial stretch, and increases resistance to flow. The result is directly seen in the aortic blood flow profile depicted by high-resistance spectral waveforms (Figure 5.3). Brain, as a low-resistance system, is able to accommodate the diastolic pressure drop through vasodilation and, as result, low-resistance waveforms appear in the precerebral and cerebral vessels (Figure 5.3). Further relationship between the electric phases of the cardiac cycle and a normal MCA spectral waveform is shown in Figure 5.4.

The electrical initiation of systole (R–S) precedes the arrival of the peak systolic complex in the MCA (Figure 5.4). The systolic upstroke is sharp if the heart valves and vessels proximal to the sampling point are normal and patent. Once blood volume is ejected by the heart (also known as the stroke volume), it enters the arterial system at changing pressures from the systolic (maximum) to diastolic (minimum) pressures. The arterial system therefore acts as a pressure reservoir capable of converting different pressures created by the heart into a relatively constant flow, particularly through parenchymal organs such as brain (remember the abovementioned Windkessel effect).

For any flow to occur, there should be a **pressure gradient** between the beginning and the end of a vessel or across the connector between two circulatory systems. This pressure gradient determines normal blood flow distribution as well as recruitment of collaterals, flow diversion, and hemodynamic steal phenomena, which will be discussed in detail in subsequent chapters.

Blood pressure (BP) parameters are used to describe systemic circulatory conditions. Because the arterial system maintains antegrade flow despite the ups and downs of pressure during the cardiac cycle, **mean arterial pressure** (MAP) is a more reliable marker of systemic arterial pressure. A practical way of determining MAP is as follows:

$$\text{MAP} = [(\text{systolic pressure} - \text{diastolic pressure})/3] + \text{diastolic pressure}$$

A simple way to remember this is: MAP (as well as the mean flow velocity) is two-thirds less than the peak systole to end diastole.

Another parameter is the **pulse pressure**, that is the difference between the peak systolic and end diastolic pressures. Pulse pressure is a marker of arterial capacitance. Because normal systolic and diastolic BP values are 120/70 mmHg, it appears that a normal pulse pressure should be about 50 mmHg. Interestingly, a normal response of brain vasculature to a drop in systemic pressure or cardiac output is to vasodilate, whereas the systemic circulation meets this challenge with vasoconstriction to maintain intravascular pressure. Thus, brain is able to continue receiving blood flow even if the BP is low. Chronic conditions, like atherosclerosis and hypertension, increase pulse pressure and reduce arterial compliance. This, in turn, creates more workload for the heart (also known as the **afterload**), and an increase in the ejected stroke volume of blood. Cardiogenic or hypovolemic shock conditions produce an opposite effect: decreased and

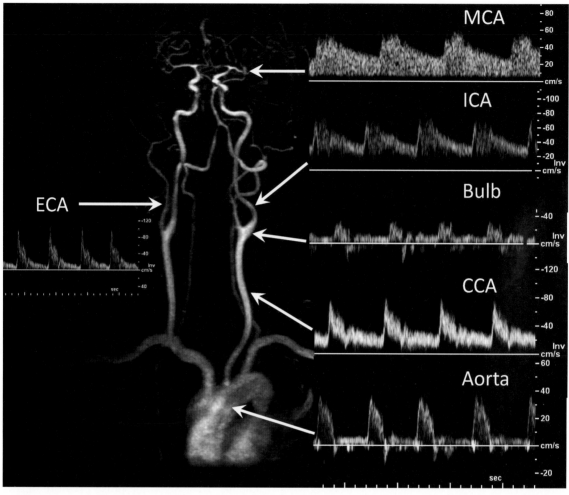

Figure 5.3 The cardiac cycle and resulting middle cerebral artery spectral waveform. CCA, common carotid artery; ECA, external carotid artery; ICA, internal carotid artery; MCA, middle cerebral artery; .

narrowed pulse pressures from a decrease in cardiac output. In septic shock, the pulse pressure can be higher and wider due to peripheral vasodilation.

As blood leaves the aorta and its large branches, the vessels continue to divide and diminish in caliber. From a very pulsatile (or high-resistance) aortic flow profile, brain is able to extract continuous low-resistance flow throughout the entire cardiac cycle (Figure 5.3). The waveforms shown in Figure 5.3 were obtained in a healthy middle-aged volunteer. All waveforms in this figure have a vertical or rapid early systolic flow acceleration, implying that blood reached each vessel without delay and with no significant

blockages. The aorta has flow reversal during closure of the aortic valve and very low diastolic velocities. The common carotid artery (CCA) has signs of both high and low resistance as it supplies the external (ECA) and internal (ICA) carotid arteries. The ECA velocity rapidly decelerates to low diastolic values. Flow separation occurs in the bulb where a low-velocity waveform was obtained from the dilated portion of the vessel. The ICA and the middle cerebral artery (MCA) have a stepwise or slow flow deceleration with diastolic velocities usually comprising 25–50% of the peak systolic values. These are the signs of a low resistance to flow in the brain vasculature.

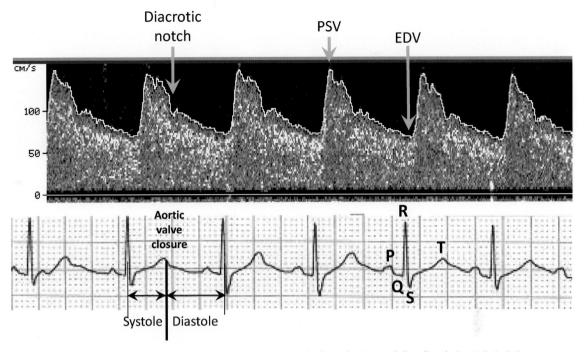

Figure 5.4 Spectral waveforms and resistance changes in the precerebral vessels. EDV, end-diastolic velocity; P, Q, R, S, T, electrocardiographic complexes; PSV, peak systolic velocity. Systole occupies approximately one-third of the cycle while the rest belongs to diastole, which starts at the diacrotic notch or the aortic valve closure. See text for the explanation.

Along this pathway from the heart to the brain, the arterial wall undergoes structural changes from purely elastic vessels, such as the aortic arch and the CCA, to the more muscular component which is present in the ICA and MCA towards arterioles and precapillary sphincters. Arterioles and sphincters act as the gate keepers and regulate the brain blood flow volume with much efficiency. This is accomplished through dilation and constriction of these vessels, which modulate capillary filling to match the metabolic needs of a specific brain region.

The easiest way to see the speed and magnitude of flow adjustment by these vessels is to change carbon dioxide blood levels through voluntary hyperventilation and breath-holding (Figure 5.5). **Breath-holding** raises CO_2 levels in blood, inducing vasodilation and increasing the blood flow volume. **Hyperventilation** reduces CO_2 levels in blood, leading to vasoconstriction and a decrease in the blood flow. Spectral waveforms reflect these processes through changes in velocity and pulsatility. However, velocity cannot be equated with flow volume because the diameter of the insonated

intracranial artery remains unknown at the time of measurement. Changes in flow velocity are proportionate to changes in arterial blood flow volume through a particular intracranial artery only under the following conditions:

1. the angle of insonation or artery intercept remains constant;

2. systemic blood pressure and cardiac output are unchanged; and

3. the territory perfused by the intercepted artery is unchanged.

The latter becomes very important due to the anatomy and complexity of brain functions. Because arterial bifurcations become more common as vessels divide and decrease in diameter, an uncertainty raises as to the path of blood flow. Blood flow utilization depends on the metabolic demand of brain tissues, which can change with activation of specific brain regions. The process of **neurovascular coupling** is responsible for the ability of neurons to increase arterial blood inflow to meet new metabolic demands, such as seen in the posterior cerebral artery with the

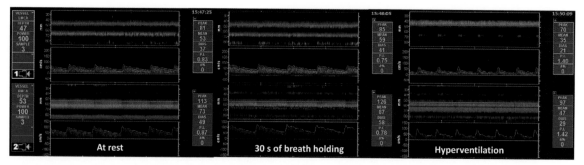

Figure 5.5 Flow velocity and pulsatility changes with breath holding for 30 seconds (measurement made at 34 seconds) and hyperventilation.

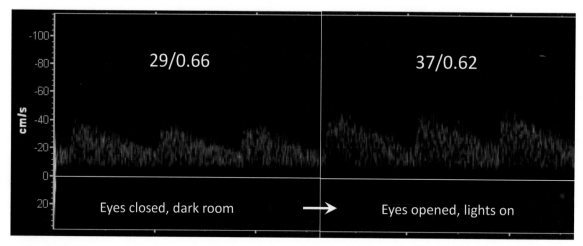

Figure 5.6 Mean flow velocity and pulsatility index changes in the posterior cerebral artery from resting to light activation.

light activation test of the visual cortex (Figure 5.6). Similar tasks can be applied to other arterial territories though with less striking results: for example open–close fist for the middle and tap-foot for the anterior cerebral arteries.

After passing through arterioles, blood reaches capillaries and delivers oxygen, nutrients, and a myriad of signaling and other important molecules to the tissues, and clears byproducts of cell functions. In- or out-of-tissue diffusion is primarily dependent on solute concentration and pressure gradients. Filtration and re-absorption across capillary walls is governed by the **Starling equilibrium**, which accounts for the interplay of the following main forces:

1. intracapillary pressure of up to 30 mmHg, a force that promotes filtration through capillary walls;

2. interstitial fluid pressure of approximately 3 mmHg, which provides for the pressure gradient that pulls fluid into the interstitial space;

3. interstitial fluid colloid osmotic pressure of approximately 8 mmHg, which promotes osmotic fluid shifts into the interstitial space; and

4. plasma colloid pressure (or oncotic pressure) of approximately 28 mmHg, which promotes capillary re-absorption.

Although the list is by no means complete, other factors can also affect the exchange of substances across the capillary wall:

1. metabolic demand (figure 5.6);

2. viscosity of the filtrate; and

3. the integrity of capillary walls (blood–brain barrier opening or breaking down).

It appears that red blood cells may not be passing through all available capillaries. Some may be inactive, some may be affected by a disease process. Assuming that a tissue is at rest, perfusion quite possibly occurs through some, but not all, available capillaries. After passing through these working capillaries, or the so-called shunts (i.e. preferential channels that connect arterioles to veins bypassing inactive capillaries), blood reaches the venous system. With tissue activation, more of these channels open, unless a disease process narrows the lumen and precludes erythrocytes from reaching the entire microvasculature.

The **venous system** is a volume reservoir of variable capacity, a collector of blood that brings it back to the heart. Often overlooked by clinicians for its significance outside of central venous thrombosis, veins offer one of the "last frontiers" for exploration in stroke patients. The closer we examine our assumptions, the more an inquisitive observer may be surprised at how much dogma dominates current thinking, and how much is overlooked.

Anyway, the right atrial pressure or **central venous pressure** (CVP) is regulated through the following main factors:

1. total blood volume;
2. the heart's ability to optimally receive and pump blood; and
3. the capacitance of the venous system.

Under normal conditions, the atmospheric pressure approximates CVP (CVP = 0). An increase in total blood volume, reduced left or right ventricular performance, or maximized venous capacitance will result in an elevated CVP.

Breathing also affects venous return. Remember that **inspiration** leads to the following:

1. increase in chest volume;
2. decrease in intrathoracic pressure;
3. increase in venous return from the arms and head;
4. downward movement of the diaphragm;
5. increase in the abdominal pressure; and
6. decrease in venous return from the legs.

Expiration produces the opposite changes:

1. decrease in chest volume;
2. increase in the intrathoracic pressure;
3. decrease in venous return from the arms and head;
4. upward movement of the diaphragm;
5. decrease in the abdominal pressure; and
6. increase in venous return from the legs.

To memorize these effects, remember the following exercise that helps athletes to improve venous return to the heart and recover faster after physical activities – with inspiration, raise both arms above the head; with expiration, drop arms and bend forward.

After reviewing the entire cycle of blood movement through the circulatory system, let's discuss the parameters used to describe systemic hemodynamic conditions.

Cardiac output (CO) represents the amount of blood that is ejected by the left ventricle into the aorta over 1 minute. The normal average CO value is 5 L/min; however, it substantially varies in adults from 4 to 8 liters according to body size. To compensate for these variations, the **cardiac index** (CI) is used to estimate the proportion of blood flow to body surface area (BSA):

CI = CO/BSA (normal CI values
    are $2.8-4.2$ L/min/m^2)

Total CO is calculated as:

Total CO = heart rate × stroke volume

Stroke volume (SV) is the amount of blood ejected from the left ventricle with each contraction. Stroke volume is calculated as the difference in:

SV = left ventricular end-diastolic volume
    – residual left ventricular blood volume

An average adult stroke volume is 60–100 mL/ventricular contraction. Note that the left ventricle is filled up to its current maximum value at the end of heart relaxation, or end-diastoli. The blood is then ejected during systoli but some volume remains in the ventricle after the closure of the aortic valve, and the latter is termed the residual left ventricular blood flow volume. In congestive heart failure (CHF), ejection fraction decreases, CV decreases, and the residual volume increases.

CO is dependent on the heart rate and factors such as preload, contractility, and afterload. **Preload** is determined by venous return as well as the overall intravascular blood flow volume. **Contractility** of the heart muscle can be compromised by stunned myocardium, myocardial infarction, congestive heart failure, etc. **Afterload** is governed by the systemic vascular resistance as well as a myriad of conditions that can affect the vasculature and the body organs.

Autoregulation of blood flow and responses to physical activity or metabolic demands throughout the body require changes in CO. To accomplish this, the heart rate and contractility must adjust from beat to beat to provide the required amounts of blood through filling the left ventricle and delivering it through subsequent ejection. The heart must respond to a variety of neurogenic, chemical, and pressure stimuli to keep up with changing body demands, including the heart's own needs. One can appreciate the dynamics of autoregulation by observing various rhythms of beat-to-beat velocity variations and adjustments that heart makes to ever-changing circulatory, breathing, and metabolic conditions in the body. The more researchers look into biochemistry and gene regulation, the more fine-tuning created by nature is being discovered.

Nevertheless, a normal adult heart rate of between 60 and 100 beats per minute is maintained through a spontaneous electrical pacemaker activity in the sinoatrial (SA) node, termed **automaticity**. A decrease in CO produces a rapid increase in the heart rate to maintain adequate systemic blood flow.

The initial increase in the heart rates decreases the left ventricular filling time, yet it is associated with an improved myocardial contractile function. This is also known as the **Treppe phenomenon**, the mechanism to deliver more blood flow within physiologic range of demands. As heart rate increases beyond a typical rhythm of the SA node mediated responses (i.e. tachycardia > 100 beats/min), the diastolic filling declines sharply and the left ventricle's contractile function also starts to drop due to its own unmet increase in metabolic demand. Remember, that the heart is perfused in diastoli (not in systoli when the muscle contracts), so a significant reduction in the diastolic time will diminish the heart's performance and decrease CO. Interestingly, athletes can push themselves to perform in the "zone" when the heart contracts frequently yet efficiently to meet challenges of fierce competition. At rest, these athletes often have very slow heart rates (ranging sometimes between 30 and 40 beats/min). This will be important to further understand cerebral blood flow pulsatility changes with the heart rate. Meanwhile, let's examine how the heart muscle loads the ventricular volume and launches the blood pool into the aorta.

The heart's performance is linked to the pressure–flow relationship, or the **Frank–Starling law**. It relates the muscle fiber lengthening to the development of tension, explaining how preload influences the resulting contractile force. As the heart chamber is filled by the incoming blood, it lengthens the left ventricular muscle fibers. Within a physiological range of pressures, the more the end diastolic volume lengthens the muscle, the greater is the amount of tension and subsequent contractile force with which blood is ejected during systole. An analogy here is an archer who wants to shoot an arrow farther: one has to bend a bow more by stretching the string to launch the arrow. However, every system has its limits for optimal function. Similar to the left heart, the performance of the right heart is affected by these factors and should be taken into account because both (right and left) circuits of circulation as well as the heart chambers are interconnected in their performance.

In other words, going back full circle leads to the statement that the product of CO and SVR is the **arterial blood pressure** (BP). Remember from earlier discussion, for any flow to occur there has to be a pressure gradient, and CO and SVR influence BP in the opposite ways (except sepsis when CO increases and SVR remains low). Commonly, when cardiac output falls due to reduced contractility or preload values, SVR will increase in an attempt to maintain BP within normal parameters. This highlights an important difference in responses of systemic and brain circulation to failing CO. While SVR is rising, brain vessels will drop their resistance further by vasodilation, thus allowing even a failing heart to perfuse brain continuously during the cardiac cycle. This is also the mechanism by which the brain gets its constant share of blood flow despite variations in the heart function or systemic conditions. It is an important concept for interpreting cerebrovascular ultrasound studies and we will be coming back to it.

This is also fundamental to understanding why BP monitoring for rapid detection of clinically significant changes is a relatively poor tool at the bedside. Remember that BP may appear normal while patients experience early clinical deterioration and declining myocardial performance because SVR increases in response to the initial reduction in contractility. In patients with acute stroke, arterial BP remains elevated during the first days and decreases over time while the damage to the brain is being completed, and it is uncertain if higher BP values can maintain collateral flow. Understanding cardiac function, systemic conditions, severity of arterial obstruction, residual flow, and conditions distal of the proximal occlusion are keys to further advances in reperfusion therapies. The development of new, collateral flow augmentation, tissue oxygen driven, and microcirculation-assessment-based approaches to stroke treatment are eagerly awaited.

Returning to our examination of hemodynamics, SVR can be calculated if the following variables are known: mean arterial pressure (MAP), right atrial pressure (RAP or CVP), and CO:

$$SVR = [(MAP - RAP) \times 80]/CO$$

Attempts to understand BP and manage it in acute stroke patients should be linked to active monitoring of systemic hemodynamics with more sophisticated tools that analyze cerebral blood flow together with heart function and SVR. Neuroendocrine regulation and pharmacological interventions to achieve these goals are beyond the scope of this chapter and can be found elsewhere. The focus here will be on the simple tools available to a clinician for assessment of cerebral blood flow, and how to identify and differentiate certain normal and pathological responses of the cerebral vasculature.

Sampling blood flow parameters in real time is one of the key advantages of ultrasound. Even though the so-called "luminograms", that is catheter or CT/MR-based angiography, captured clinicians attention and trust in treatment decision making, ultrasound provides physiological information that is complimentary and often superior to a simplistic snap-shot image of a reduction in the vessel diameter. The main disadvantage of ultrasound has been its extreme operator dependency, not only in the quality of data acquisition (i.e. scanning) but also in its interpretation particularly for the intracranial vessels. As described in the previous chapter, transcranial Doppler is a very basic ultrasound technology which turned out to be one of the most difficult and complex tests in vascular medicine in terms of performance and interpretation skills. Carotid duplex offers far more complex technology for vessel interrogation and more straightforward diagnostic criteria, yet even these skills require continuous

education and numerous courses for health professionals worldwide to master the basics of cerebrovascular ultrasound testing. So, should we not even try to grasp ultrasound methods? I think to the contrary. We should be making much more rapid progress than we are currently in understanding the beat-to-beat physiology, as the opportunities to unveil how the body works in real time are increasing with the available tools to diagnose, correct, or prevent its malfunction.

Learning the principles of hemodynamics and mastering the tools of its assessment should be a mandatory part of the education of health professionals involved in the diagnosis and treatment of cerebrovascular diseases. Neurology residents have that startled look on their face once I begin telling them about the cardiac cycle, resistance, and brain vasculature responses to various stimuli. Yet this information enables clinicians eager to learn about body functions to navigate through differential diagnosis, understand disease progression, and individualize treatment options beyond the degree of stenosis or a certain antiplatelet strategy when dealing with a complex and dynamic process such as stroke.

Now, back to the physics of flow assessment. Information about flow dynamics can be obtained with continuous or pulsed wave ultrasound techniques. Because the latest technologies offer image-guided Doppler sampling of blood flow or multidepth Doppler gate placement, assessment of precerebral vessels with continuous wave Doppler is no longer recommended. The main reason is that there is no depth discrimination with CW Doppler and no imaging can be obtained with this technique.

A transducer emits ultrasound at a certain transmitted frequency, which for vascular investigations ranges from 1 MHz to 10 MHz. Commonly, TCD devices use 2 MHz (some have 1 MHz and 1.6 MHz probes); transcranial duplex is generally performed with 2–4 MHz dual frequency probes with lower frequencies used for Doppler sampling; and carotid duplex ranges from 4 MHz to 12 MHz with most Doppler sampling done at 4–7 MHz frequencies.

After an ultrasound beam encounters a moving object, the transmitted frequency can be modified, as shown in Figure 5.7. Baseline (horizontal axis) indicates the transmitted frequency and no frequency shift is seen with vessel intercept at 90 degrees.

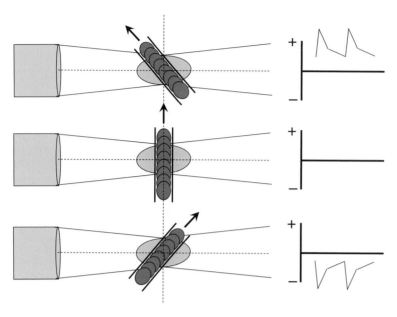

Figure 5.7 Returned frequency shifts. Positive, absent, or negative Doppler shits from the transmitted frequency are determined by the angle of interception of the vessel (<90, 90, and >90 degrees respectively). In other words, red blood cells moving (arrow) towards the probe will increase the returned frequency, and those moving away will decrease the frequency relative to the emitted value.

With TCD, the emitted frequency is 2 MHz, well above the audible range. The Doppler shift induced by moving blood ranges from 20 to 20 kHz, and these frequencies comprise the audible output. The process that separates the shifted echoes from the emitted frequency is called **demodulation**.

Doppler shift represents the following difference:

Doppler shift (Hz) = reflected frequency

– transmitted frequency

The shift in frequency is proportionate to blood flow velocity. It is important to understand the difference between speed and velocity. Speed reflects how fast the object is moving. Velocity describes how fast and in which direction the movement occurs. Because Doppler shift is related to blood flow velocity and the angle of flow interception, the Doppler equation becomes:

Doppler shift = 2 × speed of blood × transducer

frequency × cos Θ/propagation speed

where cos Θ is the cosine function of a Doppler angle, and 2 is a coefficient that refers to two Doppler shifts (one occurs at ultrasound intercept of moving blood cells and the second one at the beam return to the transducer surface).

Doppler angle is an important concept in vascular ultrasound, and the choice of **angle correction** (Figures 5.8 and 5.9) can greatly affect the resulting velocity measurements. Doppler sampling occurs within the gate represented by the two short parallel lines at the interception of lines 1 and 2 (spectral gate), and within the entire area of the box (3) (color flow imaging with colors indicating flow direction and mean frequency shifts) (Figure 5.8).

Note, it is impossible to apply proper angle correction without structural imaging (Figure 5.9). Thus, all TCD studies are done at an assumed zero degree angle of insonation. If one sets a Doppler angle above 60 degrees, this can lead to velocity overestimation and potentially false-positive results. Most carotid duplex studies and diagnostic criteria refer to velocities obtained with 45–60 degrees angle of insonation.

Angle correction can be done parallel to the flow or to the vessel walls, or both if they are parallel to each other (Figure 5.9). In experienced hands, both techniques yield results of similar accuracy in grading carotid stenosis. To optimize color image to guide spectral interrogation, not only the color box has to be angled appropriately to the vessel position and direction but also the color flow scale needs to accommodate the velocity spectrum without an artifact.

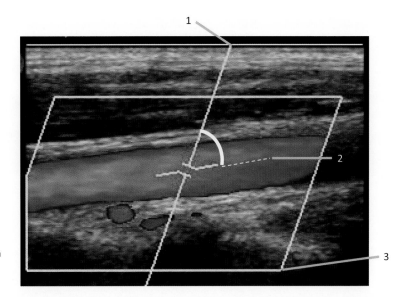

Figure 5.8 Doppler angle, steering axis, and color flow box. A color flow duplex image shows: 1, steering axis; 2, "shoulder" which should be lined up with either flow direction or vessel wall; 3, angled color flow box.

Spectral waveform analysis remains the mainstay of vascular assessment with ultrasound. Gray-scale or color flow images can be helpful and highly suggestive of a certain pathological process but the definitive conclusions are generally drawn after the waveforms are optimized and velocity measurements are obtained. Waveforms themselves also have clues to lesion localization (Figure 5.10).

If you sample a vessel, the lesion, if any, can only be located in three places: distal to the site of insonation, at the site of insonation, and proximal to the site of insonation (Figure 5.10). Key features that point to lesion location are systolic acceleration and pulsatility. With lesions distal to the site of insonation, the systolic flow acceleration remains normal and the end-diastolic velocities may decrease if this lesion is flow limiting. If a lesion is located proximal to the site of insonation, there could be a delay in systolic flow acceleration but pulsatility should remain low because this flow is going to the brain which will likely vasodilate to compensate for this lesion. If a stenosis is located at the site of insonation, one can expect a focal velocity increase proportionate to the degree of a stenosis.

The relationship between the degree of a stenosis, flow velocity, and volume has been described by Merrill P. Spencer and John M. Reid, and now known at the Spencer's curve (Figure 5.11). Spencer and Reid applied the Hagen–Poiseuille law, continuity principle, and cerebrovascular resistance to build an axis-symmetric flow model. This model has since been widely used for interpretation of cerebrovascular ultrasound studies as a means of explaining the velocity behavior with various degrees of arterial stenosis.

Several key hemodynamic principles are reflected in the curve. The Spencer's curve is a polynomial curve of the third order because the predicted arterial blood flow velocity shows both linear and nonlinear components in its rise, with a subsequent decrease to the zero level owing to the cubic function. This means that the peak systolic velocity (PSV) is inversely proportionate to several functions of the residual lumen diameter (d):

$$PSV \sim 1/d + d^2 + d^3$$

An explanation how the first and second powers of vessel diameter influence the velocity behavior is provided below. The fourth power of the vessel diameter ($d^4 = (2r)^4$, where r is the vessel radius), is also likely to play a role as it directly influences flow volume and resistance to flow. However, it is the cubic function (d^3) that really explains the turn of the curve from the up-slope down to the down-slope with the most severe vessel narrowing. Higher powers of radius may

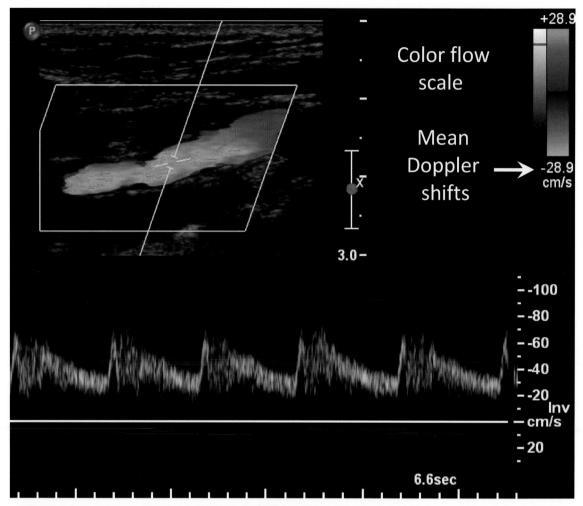

Figure 5.9 Color aliasing in a normal vessel due to low color flow scale settings. Spectral Doppler shows normal velocities in the ICA (waveform at the bottom of the image) just distal to the exit from the bulb. The waveform represents a spectrum of Doppler shift frequencies calculated using the Fast Fourier transformation (FFT). Color flow scale is set too low at 28.9 cm/s mean velocity to display flow without an artifact.

also play a role but their contribution in construction of the model is practically negligible.

Spencer and Reid built their model using a vessel with straight walls, no bifurcations, and placed an axis-symmetric and smooth-surface stenosis. In this situation, the flow velocity and cross-sectional areas (*A*) are linked in the so-called "continuity principle" until very severe grades of the stenosis that paradoxically reduce flow velocity:

$$A_1 \times PSV_1 = A_2 \times PSV_2$$

Because fluid is noncompressible and because the applied pressure remained the same in the Spencer and Reid model, the maximum stenotic (PSV_2) velocity increases by the amount inversely proportionate to the squared function of the residual vessel diameter:

$$PSV_2 = \frac{A_1 PSV_1}{A_2} \text{ or } PSV \sim \frac{1}{\pi r^2} \text{ or } \frac{1}{d^2}$$

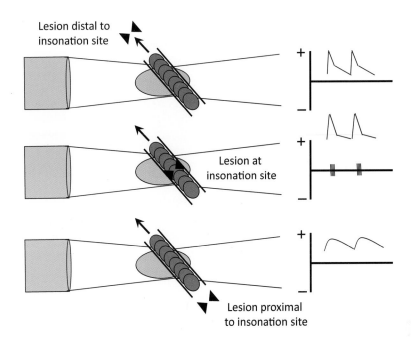

Lesion distal to insonation site

Lesion at insonation site

Lesion proximal to insonation site

Figure 5.10 Typical waveforms with lesion location relative to the site of insonation. Further explanations are in the text.

Hence, the prestenotic (PSV$_1$) velocity is not shown in the graph (Figure 5.11). However, the graph contains the initial velocity value with 0 degree stenosis, or normal vessel patency. This could be used as a reference point (or range) in subsequent estimations of disease severity by the velocity changes. Most adults will have (or had at some point) a normal ICA velocity of less than 125 cm/s (commonly 60–80 cm/s). Knowing this helped to develop thresholds for PSV increase as well as ratios. Subsequent research showed that velocity ratios could complement absolute measurements of the maximum velocity despite the presence of bifurcations.

Flow acceleration begins at the stenosis entrance where the pressure energy of flow (i.e. blood pressure) is converted into the kinetic energy, resulting in increased velocities. This conversion of energy is described by the **Bernoulli effect**:

$$P_1 - P_2 = \Delta P = \frac{1}{2}\rho(V_1^2 - V_2^2)$$

where ρ is the density of the fluid, which has not been commented on but presumably remained stable in the Spencer and Reid model. The velocity changes are therefore mainly driven by the arterial pressure (P)

gradient and the size of the residual lumen. Assuming that arterial blood pressure remained constant across various degrees of the carotid stenosis, the model showed that the initial PSV increase compensated for the flow volume through the residual lumen (Figure 5.11). Remember that velocity should not be equated with flow volume even though both are driven by the pressure gradients. Further PSV increase with severe stenoses becomes inefficient to maintain flow volume. Note that flow volume only starts to decrease at 70% but markedly drops with ≥80% stenosis (Figure 5.11). Remarkably, 70% diameter reduction in a vessel corresponds to 91% area reduction and blood still manages to mostly compensate for this reduction or degree of the stenosis. The commonly used term "hemodynamically significant" stenosis refers to a significant pressure or flow volume drop across the stenosis that prompts recruitment of collateral flow to compensate for this arterial lesion. This is an important phenomenon to remember because sometimes the velocity changes may not adequately reflect the disease severity and only indirect downstream measurements unmask the significance of the lesion. Examples include tandem stenoses (whereby moderate stenoses may impede flow to a greater extent than their simple sum) or elongated stenoses (whereby the length of the lesion

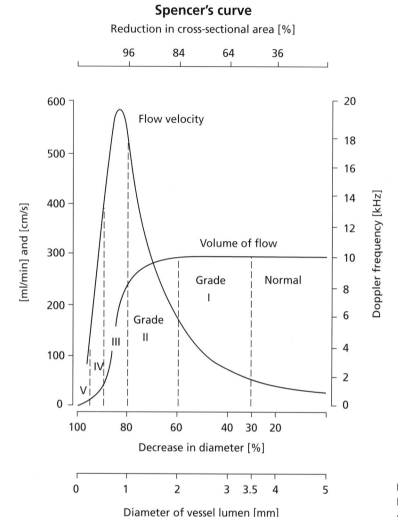

Figure 5.11 The relationship between blood flow velocity, volume, and the degree of a stenosis.

creates more resistance to flow than the actual diameter reduction). This flow volume decrease will occur particularly if the cerebrovascular resistance also does not decrease distal to a severe stenosis, as was assumed for simplicity of the model. Notably, the flow volume per unit of time directly depends on the pressure difference described in the Hagen–Poiseuille law.

In the Spencer and Reid model, no compensatory poststenotic vasodilation was introduced and the fluid viscosity as well as the length of the arterial stenosis were also assumed to remain stable. Thus, an axis-symmetric, smooth-surface, presumably short-length and circular arterial narrowing (a cerebrovascular

oxymoron!) produced, not surprisingly, a perfect correlation between the arterial flow velocity, flow volume, and increasing degree of the carotid stenosis under these controlled and ideal circumstances. The model, based on few elements, was proposed to predict the arterial flow velocity behavior across the entire spectrum of carotid stenosis, and to derive diagnostic criteria for spectral Doppler ultrasound for grading the stenosis. As you will see below, it turned out to be a good road map for interpretation of cerebrovascular ultrasound studies.

Application of hemodynamic principles to interpretation of vascular ultrasound studies is a complex task, which requires careful clinical and pathophysiological considerations. In reality, most arterial stenoses are axis-asymmetric with irregular surface, and have variable lesion length and compliance of the vessel wall, not to mention bilateral lesions. The blood viscosity, pressure, and distal resistance also vary between patients and within an individual over time. Therefore, the Spencer's curve could best serve as a guide rather then a source of actual velocity values for grading an arterial stenosis. However, the model reflected the general direction of hemodynamic changes with carotid disease and it has survived the test of time as a basis to explain individual hemodynamic changes and to understand the results of clinical research.

To interpret any given blood flow velocity value obtained in a patient, one must consider whether this velocity was found on the up-slope, on the down-slope, or "the other side" of the Spencer's curve. For example, an abnormally elevated flow velocity is most likely to be found on the up-slope of the Spencer's curve, that is within the 50–90% ICA diameter reduction range. How can one decide if a given velocity is abnormal? If there is a reference velocity value, such as mid-to-distal CCA or an unobstructed ICA before the stenosis or on the contralateral side, an arterial stenosis of about 50% diameter reduction will double the velocity value assumed normal for a particular patient. Because the ICA has a bulb that normally has low velocities and could be affected by an axis-asymmetric plaque, the CCA velocity and the ICA/CCA PSV ratios were introduced to compensate for this clinical uncertainty. Remember that in a vessel with straight walls and a focal single lesion:

50% stenosis *doubles* the velocity; and
70% stenosis *quadruples* the velocity.

Despite wide interindividual variations, the peak systolic velocity itself remains the single best predictor of a focal stenosis severity. When PSV exceeds 125 cm/s, one can say with a great degree of certainty that a patient with an atheroma has a ≥50% ICA stenosis (if the area of the stenosis is short, if this patient is also free of abnormal systemic hemodynamic changes, etc.: this list of if's can go on and on). However, the same velocity thresholds should not be applied for carotid arteries that have been stented, or bear tandem lesions, or if a distal or contralateral occlusion is present. This, as well as a multiparametric

approach to grading carotid stenosis and other lesions, will be discussed later in the book.

To add to confusion, elevated, "normal" and decreased velocities can also be found on the "other side" of the Spencer's curve, that is with the so-called angiographic "string" signs or near-occlusions indicating most severe arterial stenoses. The differential diagnosis prompts the use of multifactorial criteria, that is the velocity ratios between the prestenotic and stenotic segments (i.e. the ICA/CCA PSV ratios), velocity asymmetry between homologous segments on bilateral examinations, B-mode imaging, color or power flow and spectral waveform analyses, and downstream poststenotic flow changes and collateral assessment. The latter in particular becomes important because lesions "on the other side" of the Spencer's curve are almost always hemodymanically significant, producing flow volume decrease and pressure drop across the lesion, which create the demand to recruit downstream collaterals. All these factors should be considered when a patient with stroke is evaluated in the emergency room or a patient with transient ischemic attack and a carotid near-occlusion walks into an outpatient clinic. If stroke severity is less than expected for a proximal lesion location or the patient is currently symptom free, this means that somehow his or her circulation is maintaining cerebral blood flow and avoiding devastating, or even detectable, neurological deficit.

Figure 5.12 illustrates changes in proximal intracranial arterial waveforms to compensate for an arterial obstruction. Note, the brain is able to maintain a low-resistance circulatory bed and the waveforms represent still favorable perfusion conditions because the patient remained asymptomatic despite progression of the arterial steno-occlusive disease in the proximal left ICA. Specific compensatory changes are seen as follows:

1. a right-to-left partial anterior cross-filling (right A1 ACA MFV > MCA, turbulent disturbed flow signal from likely hypoplastic or stenotic left A1 ACA which appears reversed);

2. a blunted left M1 MCA spectral waveform (despite clearly delayed systolic flow acceleration, MCA still shows a low resistance flow indicating that it is a post-obstructive flow into a vascular bed with low resistance, i.e. vasodilation);

3. the left PCommA or P1 PCA flow signal towards the probe has the systolic flow acceleration better than

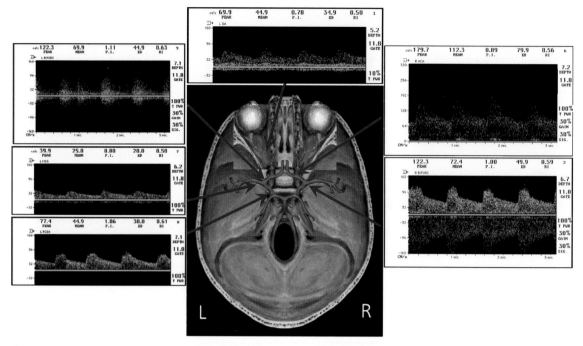

Figure 5.12 Typical waveform changes on TCD in the presence of a hemodynamically significant lesion in the proximal ICA. L is left (affected) side; R is right (nonaffected) side. Bifurcation denotes spectral waveforms obtained at the terminal ICA bifurcation into the MCA above and ACA below the baseline; RACA shows an inverted spectral waveform with velocity/ pulsatility measurements for comparison with the RMCA. OA, ophthalmic artery; PComA, posterior communicating artery.

the left M1 MCA and higher MFV (finding suggesting of collateral flow via left PCommA or compensatory flow increase via left PCA indicating transcortical collateralization of flow); and

4. the reversed left OA flow – note low resistance of a truly reversed OA flow – this finding points to the proximal ICA below the OA origin as the location of a hemodynamically significant obstruction, and it also points to likely incomplete circle of Willis or insufficient collateralization via the circle intracranially.

Because the brain is metabolically dependent on a continuous supply of oxygen and glucose, the symptom-free state means that the minimum amount of nutrients necessary for function is being delivered. In my experience, patients who sustain low-resistance continuous flow even at mean flow velocities of 20 cm/s (2 MHz, assumed zero degree angle), or short-term reductions to even below this velocity, are able to get through the acute phase, sometimes even without a residual deficit. This balance, however, can be fragile indeed.

Of note, normally brain is perfused at a rate of approximately 750 mL of blood per minute from all four major precerebral vessels, or 15% of the total CO. This volume (or filling of the capacitance vessels over time) varies with age, viscosity, and heart function, as well as re-wiring of the circulation if an arterial blockage exists. However, one must remember that velocity measured by TCD or duplex cannot be equated with the blood flow volume as with current technology we do not know the area of the vessel lumen at the place of the velocity measurements. Further confounding factors include multiple intracranial bifurcations that can mask the presence of a distal lesion by low resistance/ good velocity findings in the proximal vessel, and unavoidable changes in the angle of insonation between two hand-held attempts to insonate the same vessel.

Despite these measurement limitations, sonographers and interpreting physicians need to know that resting **cerebral blood flow** (CBF) is relatively stable despite changes in cardiac output, body position, and arterial blood pressure; and in a healthy adult it amounts to approximately >50 mL/100 g of brain tissue per minute (though deceasing with age, CBF values of 80–70 mL/100 g are expected before any malfunction may occur). Under normal circumstances, focal changes in CBF correlate with metabolic demands, such as activity in a specific brain region. Corresponding changes on TCD can be captured over a short period of time during continuous monitoring at a stable angle of insonation during light activation of the PCA territory (Figure 5.6). When autoregulatory processes are functional, the brain is capable of producing varying levels of arterial perfusion pressures across a wide range of systemic arterial pressures. Higher BP or CO will result in arterioles "clamping down" on the incoming flow, thus increasing waveform pulsatility. When autoregulation is dysfunctional, brain perfusion pressures become dependent on systemic hemodynamic flow parameters. This is particularly evident with passive changes in the residual or poststenotic intracranial flow velocities during lowering of the head-of-bed from 30 degrees to flat or even −15 degrees, or in cases of the so-called reversed Robin Hood syndrome (this will be discussed in greater detail in other chapters). With the latter, the velocity changes on TCD are often accompanied by focal neurological worsening in acute stroke patients.

Further understanding of CBF, and other factors that could affect ultrasound findings, requires knowledge of the **Monro–Kellie hypothesis**. Originally postulated in the 1800s, it refers to the relationship between the confined and unchangeable size of the skull and the pressure dynamics of its contents. The skull volume is defined by bone synostosis and is rather constant through adult life. Intracranial contents, such as brain tissue, blood pool, and cerebrospinal fluid, have to interact dynamically to accommodate each other within the confined space. Each exerts a constant pressure and, because the skull itself is incapable of expanding in size, changes in the volume of any one of the intracranial contents requires a compensatory change in the volume of another. Remember that cerebrospinal fluid (CSF) is comprised largely of water, thus it is "noncompressible" within the range of physical conditions in the living organism.

Under physiological conditions, the dynamic interaction between the intracranial contents demonstrates compliance and ensures constancy of **intracranial pressures** (ICP) within the normal parameters of 0–15 mmHg. The lack of skeletal muscles within the intracranial cavity, the correct amount of CSF, and plentiful drainage make the brain a low-pressure and low-resistance system.

In a situation where CSF has no further escape and its production continues, hydrocephalus can develop, leading to an elevated ICP. An analogy here is "slamming on brakes": when a driver presses on the brake pedal, the brake fluid being noncompressible effectively transmits this pressure to break pads, and the car slows down. When ICP is elevated, the brain's resistance to flow also increases. This, in turn, requires adjustments in the systemic hemodynamic parameters ensure brain tissue perfusion, that is determining optimal cerebral perfusion pressure or maintaining the appropriate level of tissue oxygenation. As our tools for understanding, monitoring, and manipulating hemodynamics improve, the real-time physiological assessment will become increasingly important in tailoring patient management.

Before this can be achieved, stetting MAP goals and direct measurements of ICP remain center stage in managing the neurocritical care of patients. While noninvasive technologies of ICP measurements are being developed, clinical decision making relies upon direct ICP measurements with intraventricular catheters. Because the ventricles are fluid-filled reservoirs, transmission of intraventricular pressure waveforms to bedside monitoring systems reflects ICP dynamics (Figure 5.13).

Under normal compliance, the ventricular waveform transmits all phases of ventricular systole: isovolumetric contraction, rapid ventricular ejection, reduced ventricular ejection, and ventricular diastole. The intraventricular monitor shows a waveform with easy-to-recognize landmark **pressure points (P_1, P_2, P_3)** which reflect the above-mentioned parts of the cardiac cycle:

P_1 is the percussion wave and relates to the point of peak systolic pressure.

P_2 is the tidal wave and relates to the reduced systolic ejection phase of the cardiac cycle on an arterial waveform, terminating in the dicrotic notch. P_2 is used to reflect intracranial arterial autoregulation of flow in that a progressive upward movement of P_2 towards P_1, or complete loss of P_2, indicates reduced arterial compliance.

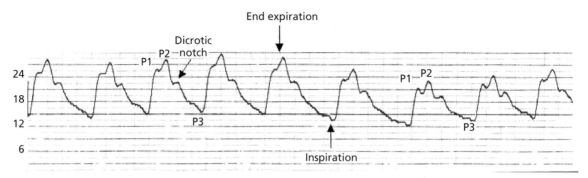

Figure 5.13 Intracranial pressure (ICP) waveform. ICP waveforms change with respiratory cycle; note the drop in pressure due to decreased cardiac output during the inspiratory phase. Unlike thoracic pressures, which fluctuate artificially with intrathoracic respiratory pressure changes, measurement at end-expiration is not used in the calculation of ICP, as both inspiratory and expiratory pressures reflect actual pressures generated within the cranial which vary with fluctuations in cardiac output. P1, peak systolic pressure; P2, tidal wave; P3, end-diastolic pressure. Note: ICP is measured at the point of P2; inspiratory and expiratory P2 measurements are averaged; ICP = 26 mmHg.

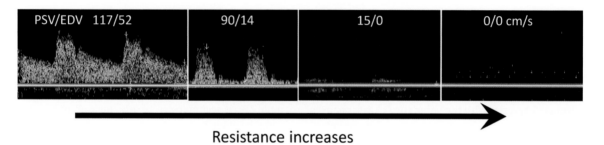

Figure 5.14 Typical waveform changes with increasing distal resistance to flow.

P_3 occurs following the dicrotic notch on the arterial waveform, that is the closure of the aortic valve and the onset of ventricular diastole.

Additional ICP modulations are affected by end-expiration or inspiration, as shown in Figure 5.13 with ICP measurements derived from P_2 points averaged between end-expiration and inspiration.

Cerebral perfusion pressure (CPP) reflects the difference in arterial inflow and venous outflow. Therefore, mean venous pressure (MVP) should be subtracted from MAP. If one assumes that ICP represents an effective closing pressure of the intracranial venous outflow system, CPP can be calculated by ICP substitution for MVP as the chief resistance factor:

$$CPP = MAP - ICP$$

Optimal CPP is defined as a pressure greater than or equal to 70 mmHg. If intracranial arterioles are able to respond, the reduction in CPP produces compensatory vasodilation. Increased stiffness in the system, overproduction of CSF with lack of its drainage, and malperfusion insults to the brain tissue can disrupt this process. Further increase in ICP can impede incoming flow and results in changes in the proximal MCA waveform morphology which can be quantified and provide rapid bedside diagnostic information if the pre-ICP increase MCA waveform was established at baseline (i.e. available for comparison with new findings) and other systemic factors like hyperventilation or increased CO were ruled out. Figure 5.14 demonstrates changes in the MCA waveforms with increasing resistance to flow. Similar changes are induced by either external compression of vasculature like with increased ICP or intravascular obstructions distal to the site of flow sampling: the first flow component to be affected is the end-diastoli (lower incoming pressure) and, as a result, waveform conversion into a high-resistance pattern with subsequent disappearance of the end-diastoli and ultimately peak systoli when resistance overwhelms the incoming flow pressure.

Spectral waveforms of the incoming flow through the proximal vessels of the circle of Willis contain a wealth of information. This is our first attempt to decipher how brain perfusion is accomplished on a beat-to-beat basis in real time, and, no doubt, much further work and some surprises lie ahead.

Recommended Reading

Hall JE. *Guyton and Hall Textbook of Medical Physiology*, 12th edn. Saunders/ Elsevier, 2010.

Journal for Vascular Ultrasound special issues on waveforms December 2011 and June 2012.

Current study materials for Vascular Technology and Interpretation offered by Davies Publishing. http://www.daviespublishing.com.

6   Real-Time Ultrasound Measures

"Measure seven times, cut once."

Russian proverb

Interpretation of ultrasound findings starts with observing real-time duplex images or multidepth motion mode displays, and continues with spectral analysis of blood flow waveforms. In the case of nonimage-guided Doppler insonation, interpretation starts with hearing the sound of blood flow, optimizing the waveform, and documenting a representative sample. It is very important to be consistent in how you perform an ultrasound test. Sonographers should use standardized scanning protocols (examples can be found in *Cerebrovascular Ultrasound in Stroke Prevention and Treatment* [1] or elsewhere in the literature [2–5]) as this will help you to learn proper techniques and identify systematic sources of error.

This chapter will describe practical parameters measured by ultrasound in real time. It is not intended to be a complete reference guide for everything that can be measured. It provides a sequence of simple measurements that I document and use to interpret sonographic findings in day-to-day practice. These measurements form the basis for the application of currently accepted diagnostic criteria as well as the differential diagnosis of vascular problems, which can be quite complex. Knowledge of the shortcomings of these measurements will help identify situations where current ultrasound technologies could offer a false result or where interrogation should be expanded with newer methods or alternative imaging techniques. Real-time ultrasound measurements are complimentary to current snap-shot structural imaging techniques.

Carotid and vertebral duplex

Visualization of living tissues on real-time imaging provides the first samples for measurements. B-mode measures include visual assessment of **echogenicity** or the echo amplitude returned from reflecting tissues. Echogenicity of moving blood is the lowest because red blood cells are weak reflectors, and the image needs to be optimized so that the vessel lumen is dark but not under-gained (Figure 6.1). The far wall of the common carotid artery (CCA) then yields better reflections from the intima, followed by media (dark layer), and then adventitia, the brightest component of the vessel wall on B-mode (Figure 6.1).

During the cardiac cycle, the vessel wall extends in systoli and decreases in size with diastoli (Figure 6.1). This process can be captured by storing a loop or real-time images, which current scanners are capable of doing. Although quantitative **distensibility** measurements are not routinely obtained, a visual inspection of the vessel wall components and motion during the cardiac cycle is one of the first parameters that I look at during extracranial carotid duplex examination. Distensibility decreases with vessel stiffening and in the presence of what looks like an occlusion; it may help to suspect chronic (no distensibility) versus acute (some distensibility or vessel wall pulsations seen in systoli) occlusion.

I further note if the **intima-media thickness (IMT)** (Figure 6.1) is greater than 1 mm (definitely abnormal thickening) and if it is greater than 1.89 mm (value in the ICA that can help reclassify patients with low or moderate Framingham Risk Score (FRS) into

Neurovascular Examination: The Rapid Evaluation of Stroke Patients Using Ultrasound Waveform Interpretation, First Edition.
Andrei V. Alexandrov.

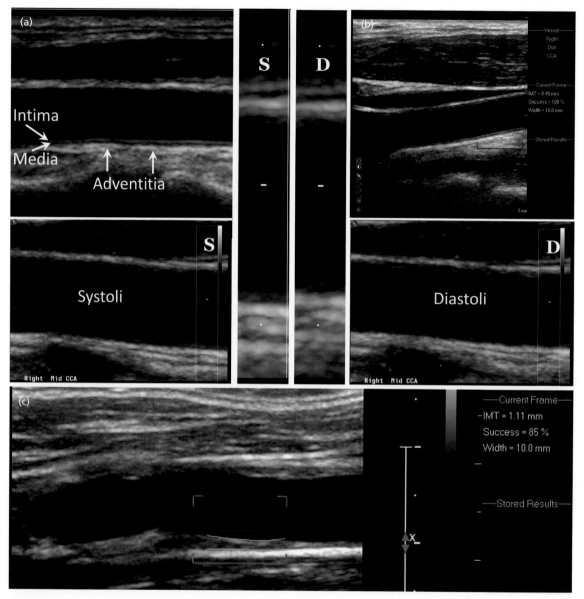

Figure 6.1 B-mode measurements of the carotid artery wall structures, pulsations, and thickness. (**a, b**) Normal appearance of intima and media thickness (IMT). S corresponds to systoli and D to diastoli appearances of the normal CCA pulsations, reflecting its distensibility. (**c**) Abnormally think IMT (1.1 mm) and early plaque formation distal to the measurement.

a high FRS category for subsequent cardiovascular events) [6]. Special software packages to measure distensibility and IMT are available and are undergoing further improvement. At the moment, I rely on visual inspection of distensibility, that is out- and inward

vessel wall motion from systoli to diastoli, and tracer measurements of best-visualized IMT segment to confirm that the IMT is thickened.

Although limited to the scanning area underneath the transducer and vessel depth, B-mode imaging can detect atherosclerosis in the carotid arteries with superb resolution [7]. An **atherosclerotic plaque** is displayed on B-mode as either a bright (echogenic or hyperechoic), mixed, or dark (echolucent or hypoechoic) structure (Figure 6.2). Shadowing, as discussed before, disturbs visualization of tissues beneath a bright reflector, and implies calcification within the plaque. **Hyperechoic** structures reflect more organized and presumably stable parts of the plaque that are more fibrous, while mixed or **hypoechoic** plaques have more cholesterol deposition, inflammation, possible intraplaque hemorrhages, and thrombi attached to the exposed core secondary to plaque rupture or ulceration [7]. Ultrasound measurements that characterize an atherosclerotic plaque describe the following:

1. plaque presence,
2. anatomic location,
3. extent,
4. texture, and
5. surface.

I judge plaque echogenicity (hyperechoic, or bright; hypoechoic or echo-lucent; and mixed) and surface (smooth vs. irregular) by visual inspection of the B-mode image. When documenting plaque extent, I always comment on whether the distal end of the plaque was successfully visualized (information of importance to a surgeon planning an operation based on carotid duplex results).

Gray-scale median and other quantitative techniques to assign a numeric value to plaque echogenicity are available but are more time consuming and are deployed mostly in research. A practical way to decide upon echogenicity is to compare plaque echoes to intima reflections: darker-then-intima parts imply echolucency while those closer to adventitia are echogenic. Plaques that are dark (at times as dark as the moving blood) are called hypoechoic and probably represent the softest and most vulnerable atherosclerotic lesions [8]. Unmasking these lesions often requires careful visual inspection of B-mode, proper gain adjustments (do not under-gain), followed by application of some form of flow imaging without changing the position of a transducer (Figures 6.3 and 6.4).

To measure plaque extent, some labs encourage actual distance measurements in the longest projections of the plaque in different planes (Figure 6.3a). Other labs, like mine, store the most representative

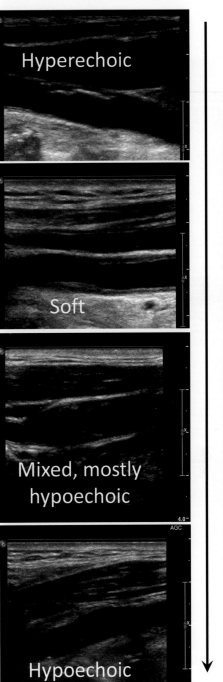

Figure 6.2 Types of plaques by echogenicity and echolucency.

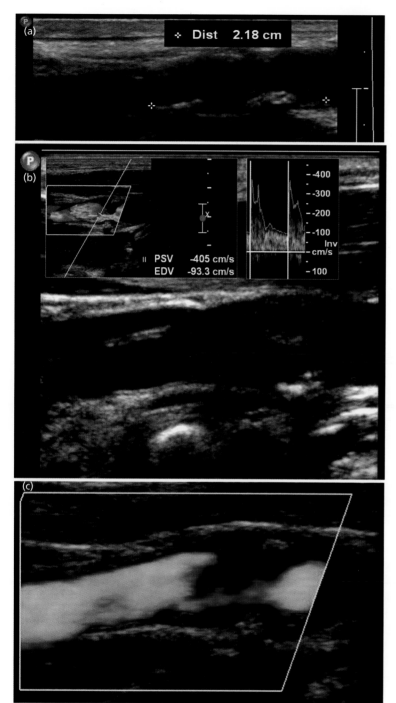

Figure 6.3 B-mode measurements plaque length and visual inspection for <50% or ≥50% stenosis. (**a**) A long (>2 cm) and less than 50% stenosing plaque. (**b**) B-mode appearance of ≥50% stenosing plaque on B-mode with corresponding power mode flow appearance (**c**), and angle corrected velocity measurements from a color flow guided image (**b** insert).

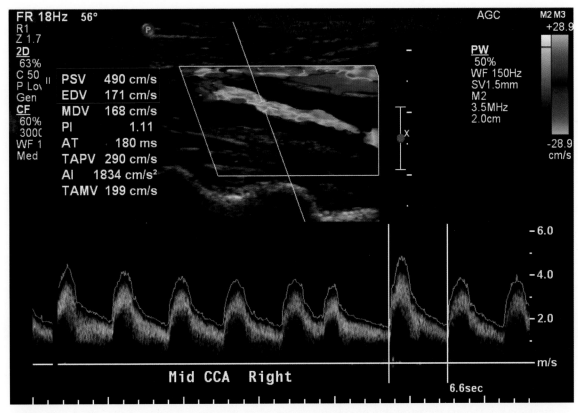

Figure 6.4 Color flow imaging unmasks a hypoechoic plaque. The stenotic lumen identifies a long (>>2 cm) hypoechoic plaque in the mid-CCA extending beyond the current field of view. This finding is of importance for planning carotid endarterectomy or stenting.

longitudinal and transverse images with and without color flow (Figure 6.3b,c) to visually inspect the plaque and quickly determine if it is:

1. <50% or ≥50% diameter-reducing lesion;

2. more or less than 2 cm long;

3. originating and particularly ending within the reach of the duplex scanning field.

These simple visual assessments are useful to later decide if:

1. the velocity increase matches the reduction of the vessel lumen (Figure 6.3, insert);

2. the plaque is too long and therefore may not produce jets expected from its maximal diameter narrowing; and

3. plaque extends beyond the duplex transducer reach, which may pose a problem for surgical exposure and clamping of the ICA during endarterectomy (because the distal end of vessel visualization on

B-mode on the left side of the image is limited by the jaw and corresponds to the vessel extent available for surgical exposure).

It could also be important for both surgeons and interventionalists to know if there is a substantial plaque burden in the CCA (Figure 6.4), and if there are tandem proximal lesions, or lesions extending beyond the surgical field on the neck.

The next step is application of color flow or power-mode imaging to depict moving blood. Flow-imaging modes are essential components of duplex scanning. I look for agreement between B-mode structural images and flow filling of the lumen, direction, resistance, and possible aliasing (Figure 6.3b, insert, and Figure 6.4). Although I start scanning with transverse application, first B-mode, then color flow or power mode superimposed on B-mode, I do *not* make area reduction measurements as these change from systoli to diastoli and are greatly affected by gain settings as well attenuation due to calcium, etc. Nevertheless, observing flow dynamics in real time can provide useful clues to the nature of the disease process and severity. A quick transverse sweep of the precerebral vessels on the neck with B-mode and power mode can be a fast screening test at the bedside, with ultrasound images akin to axial source images on CT-angiography or MR-angiography [9].

Color or power-mode flow imaging further guides placement of the spectral Doppler gate. Without spectral analysis, flow images should not be used to quantify the degree of an arterial stenosis as they are prone to artifacts and can be easily manipulated through velocity scale, gain settings, and box angulation, providing a great potential for an error. Having said that, an **optimized flow image** can be very helpful to discover a lesion not obviously seen on B-mode (Figure 6.4). Flow images can be helpful in overall qualitative assessment of the disease process. These images (as many as necessary) should be stored for documentation and interpretation purposes.

After an optimized duplex image is obtained, a Doppler gate is placed to complete the study with spectral analysis and quantitative measurements (Figure 6.4). An important part of this process is to listen to the flow signals, and to determine if gain and velocity scale settings are correct for the spectral waveform display. The main **spectral waveform parameters** that are measured include:

1. peak systolic velocity (PSV);
2. end-diastolic velocity (EDV);
3. mean flow velocity (MFV); and
4. pulsatility index (PI) of Gosling and King [10] or resistance index (RI) of Pourcellot [11].

For extracranial carotid duplex examinations, the emphasis is placed on PSV and EDV, whereas for transcranial Doppler measurements MFV and PI or RI are more commonly documented.

$$MFV = (PSV + 2EDV)/3$$

$$PI = (PSV - EDV)/MFV$$

$$RI = (PSV - EDV)/EDV$$

Additional parameters that can be measured include (Figure 6.4):

1. temporal average peak velocity (TAPV);
2. mean average diastolic velocity (MADV);
3. acceleration time (AT), in milliseconds (ms);
4. acceleration index (AI), cm/s^2;
5. temporal average mean flow velocity (TAMV);
6. flow volume (mL/min), if the vessel diameter is known (Figure 6.5).

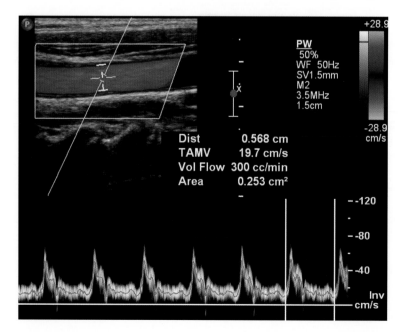

Figure 6.5 Flow volume measurements in the CCA. In this example, the CCA flow volume = 300 cc/min.

I do not use these additional parameters in routine carotid/ vertebral duplex imaging. I use the ICA/CCA PSV ratio (described below) as a way to ascertain the severity of stenosis and possible contribution of flow collateralization as well as a "poor man's substitute" for the flow volume measurements [12, 13]. Current scanners have the ability to measure flow volume (most reliably in the CCA, Figure 6.5), which may have a role in longitudinal measurements in the patient, or to unmask a flow-limiting lesion or collateralization.

As to the "bare minimum" measurements, the following **extracranial segments** should be assessed and representative B-mode ± flow imaging and spectral waveforms should be stored:

1. proximal CCA,
2. mid-to-distal CCA,
3. bulb,
4. proximal ICA,
5. most distal aspect of the ICA on the neck,
6. ECA,
7. proximal VA, preferably at its origin,
8. mid-to-distal cervical VA.

If abnormalities are found, additional segmental assessments should be documented because the assessment of the extent and severity of disease rely on the completeness of scanning examinations.

In addition to the peak systolic and end-diastolic velocities, an **ICA/CCA PSV ratio** is calculated. The ratio is between the highest PSV found anywhere along the ICA stenosis, and the mid-to-distal portion of the CCA, usually 2–4 cm below the bifurcation. To achieve consistency in where to sample the CCA, I take advantage of the fact that, regardless of the manufacturer, the length (or footprint) of linear vascular transducers for carotid imaging is quite consistent. This means that if one places the flow divider on the left side of the image and samples CCA to the right (Figure 6.6), the same CCA segment can be assessed over time. This becomes useful in follow-up because our sonographers use the patient as his or her own control with a clearly identifiable landmark. Interestingly, the length of the transducer allows sampling of the CCA 2–4 cm proximal to the bifurcation where the CCA diameter stabilizes (i.e. vessel walls become parallel) on the angiogram – an observation from the NASCET trial. Note that the ICA/CCA ratio was validated in numerous studies for this mid-to-distal loca-

tion [13], and not for the proximal segment where PSV increases due to proximity of the aorta, and the resulting ratio can be artificially low.

If a stenotic lesion is found in the CCA, I also calculate the maximum CCA stenotic PSV to the prestenotic CCA PSV ratio (Figure 6.7). As described in the previous chapter for a vessel with straight walls, a 50% diameter reduction doubles the velocity across the stenosis and a 70% stenosis quadruples the velocity [14]. If the CCA is affected by multiple or diffuse lesions, I then compare the highest velocity to the contralateral nonaffected vessel.

I calculate a similar **pre- to poststenotic PSV ratio** if a local stenosis is found in the midcervical VA. If a high-velocity jet is found at the VA origin, I calculate its maximum velocity to the poststenotic velocity ratio.

Finally, I put together visual assessment of all images, flow disturbances if any, and spectral waveform velocity data to arrive at the interpretation. I will discuss in subsequent chapters the diagnostic criteria I use and differential diagnostic algorithms.

Intracranial ultrasound

Transcranial Doppler (TCD) or transcranial color-coded duplex sonography (TCCS) aim to interrogate intracranial vessels. Regardless whether imaging, motion mode, or other modalities are deployed during scanning to depict flow, the "end result" is a vessel-segment-specific spectrogram (Figure 6.8) that measures PSV, EDV and at least two parameters are calculated from these measurements [15, 16]:

1. MFV,
2. PI (Gosling and King) or RI (Pourcellot).

One might say that this is too simplistic and I have to agree. These parameters are just the first two that we find to be useful, more so MFV than PI, at the moment. PI is regarded by many as an often misleading or imprecise reflection of the true resistance as it has limitations [17]. Other parameters describing actual blood flow await understanding and validation. Some centers use PSV and the resistance index of Pourcellot (RI) for their interpretation. Note that most current ultrasound scanners will provide measurements of PSV, EDV, MFV, PI, and RI, as well as the digital storage of echoes and postprocessed spectral

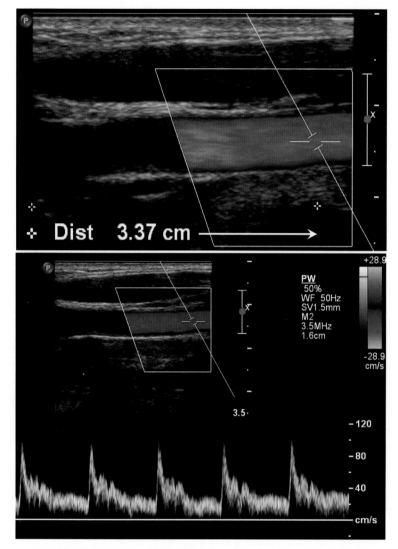

Figure 6.6 Obtaining mid-to-distal CCA peak systolic velocity measurements for calculation of the ICA/CCA PSV ratio. To achieve consistency in the position of sampling the CCA, place the flow divider to the left of the image and angle the color flow in the direction of the CCA to the right of the image. The transducer length (fairly standard between different vascular probes/ scanners used for carotid imaging) will help place the Doppler gate 2–4 cm proximal to CCA bifurcation. Distance from the flow divider is measured at 3.37 cm.

data, which allow access to all of these numbers and beyond, that is signal intensities and actual waveforms (Figure 6.8).

A duplex image can reveal vessel location, appearance, and flow direction (Figure 6.9) to help further guide spectral Doppler interrogation. These findings should be stored along with the velocity data and used for interpretation. In addition to the velocity-based measurements, intracranial examinations can reveal a variety of abnormal findings which can have diagnostic significance. Visually, an abnormal waveform can

be identified on a spectrogram [18] and these examples will be discussed in detail in a separate chapter.

With current technologies, the flow parameters should be documented for the following segments [16]:

1. proximal M1 middle cerebral artery (MCA),
2. distal M1 MCA / proximal M2 MCA,
3. A1 anterior cerebral artery (ACA),
4. P1 or P2 posterior cerebral artery (PCA),
5. terminal internal carotid artery (ICA),
6. ICA siphon,

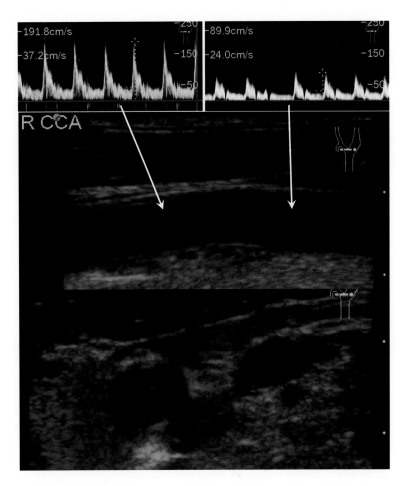

Figure 6.7 Intraluminal thrombus in the CCA causing ≥50% stenosis. B-mode shows ≥50% protrusion into the lumen and the stenotic/ prestenotic PSV ratio is ≥2.

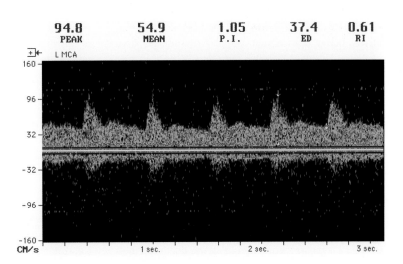

Figure 6.8 Spectral waveform and examples of intracranial flow parameter measurements. Velocity and resistance parameters are calculated from PSV and EDV measurements. Returned signal intensity is proportional to brightness of the spectra on a unicolor scale.

7. ophthalmic artery (OA),
8. terminal vertebral artery (VA),
9. proximal basilar artery (BA),
10. distal BA.

Additional measurements should be provided if any of the communicating arteries or focal lesions are found along detectable vessel segments. In patients with sub-arachnoid hemorrhage, distal ICA on the neck is also sampled with 2 MHz Doppler carrying frequency at a zero degree angle, and this value is used to calculate the so-called **Lindegaard ratio** (or **hemispheric index**) [19].

$$\text{Lindegaard ratio} = \text{maximum MFV MCA}/$$
$$\text{MFV distal unilateral ICA}$$

Normal vasculature or hyperemic changes produce a Lindegaard ratio <3, mild-to-moderate vasospasm has values 3 to less than 6, and severe vasospasm is suspected with values ≥6.

Similarly, the "modified Lindegaard index", now often called the **Soustiel index** is calculated for the basilar artery [20–22]:

$$\text{Soustiel index} = \text{maximum MFV BA}/$$
$$\text{extracranial VA MFV}$$

Normal values are below 2, mild/moderate spasm values 2–3, and severe spasm usually produces values >3. Sviri *et al.* also provided MFV thresholds to be used in combination with the Soustiel index for vasospasm prediction in the basilar artery [22].

A low MHz transcranial ultrasound (i.e. 1–2 MHz) has a unique ability to detect moving particles with impedance different from the blood [23]. It offers sensitivity better than higher Doppler frequencies used for carotid duplex Doppler sampling. Note that kHz frequencies are not used for vascular diagnostic studies. Therefore, 2 MHz TCD has become the gold standard to detect, localize, and quantify **brain embolization** in real time (Figure 6.10) [24–27]. If detected, an **embolic signal** (ES) should be properly stored and described. Ideally, its sound signature should be recorded and each component of the ES International Consensus definition [28] should be met, as listed below. Emboli have a distinct **audible component** above background flow (chirp, pop, or moaning sounds). The measurement of **intensity** above background flow should be made in decibels

(dB). The signal appearance in the fast Fourier trans-formation (FFT) processed spectral waveform should be stored to document its primary **unidirectionality**. The final measure is **randomness**. Note that ES can arrive in clusters (and the clusters could themselves be random), and this should also be documented. ES also are known in the literature as **microembolic signals** (MES) or **high-intensity transient signals** (HITS) [27, 28].

Power motion Doppler (PMD) and spectral TCD analyses can also quantify the measurements of intensity of embolic signals (ES) above concurrent blood flow. Figure 6.10 shows calculations of the **embolus-to-blood ratios** (**EBR**) for PMD display and spectral waveforms [29].

Embolic signals can occur spontaneously, originate from prosthetic heart valves, or can be detected as part of the right-to-left shunt testing and other intraoperative manipulations [30–33]. The total number of embolic signals is important for interpretation. Note, for example, the following in interpretation ". . . an ongoing brain embolization was detected at a rate of four embolic signals per minute unilateral to a proximal ICA stenosis", or when grading shunt functionality [32]. For example, less than 30 ES (or microbubbles) indicate a shunt with likely poor conductance (i.e. Spencer's grade 1 shunt [34]), which would be difficult to cross with an intracardiac catheter, whereas ≥30 ES, shower or curtain appearance of ES would indicate significant shunting (Figure 6.11).

Vasomotor reactivity (VMR) has become a useful adjunct for risk stratification, particularly with carotid artery disease [35] and in early management after stroke or transient ischemic attack [36]. It is important to distinguish between assessment of VMR (when vasodilation changes CBF), and autoregulation (which works through similar vasomotor mechanisms to maintain CBF levels at different BP values). The latter is the subject of investigations, with no uniform tech-nique currently adopted for widespread use. VMR testing, however, has gained wider acceptance and utilizes one of the three approaches [37–39]:
1. dose-controlled CO_2 inhalation,
2. diamox injection, and
3. breath-holding index.

Regardless which test is used, the measurements include baseline (or prestimulus) MFV, and MFV after a vasodilatory stimulus application for a time sufficient

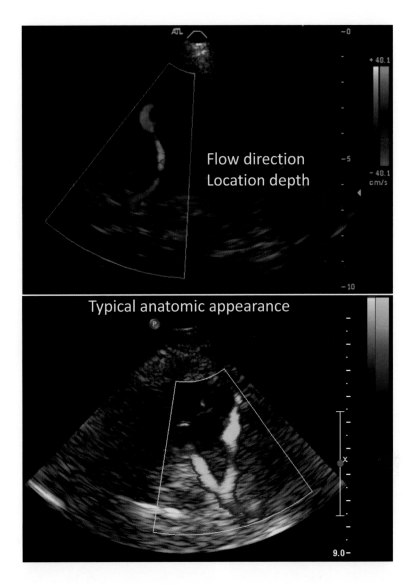

Flow direction
Location depth

Typical anatomic appearance

Figure 6.9 Transcranial duplex images. Color flow or power Doppler images superimposed on B-mode are helpful to identify vessels based on depth, appearance, and flow direction.

to induce the smooth muscle response. We assume that the given gas concentration, drug dose, or ventilatory suppression are enough to induce such a response. While an ideal challenge system is yet to emerge and measurements of oxygen consumption with positron emission tomography remain of limited access, useful clinical clues can be derived with current methods. Assessment of the intracranial circulation response is generally expressed as a percent change from baseline to poststimulus over baseline, with or without adjustment for the time it took for this response to develop.

In case of the breath-holding index (BHI) [39], it is calculated as follows (Figure 6.12):

$$BHI = [(MFV_{30s} - MFV_b)/MFV_b] \times 100/30$$
$$(\text{normal values} \geq 0.69)$$

where 30s is the number of seconds of successful breath holding (minimum 24 seconds), and b is the MFV measurement at baseline. MFV_{30s} is measured 4 seconds after the person started to breathe again. So, in a way it is MFV obtained at a range of at least 28–34 seconds after the beginning of breath holding.

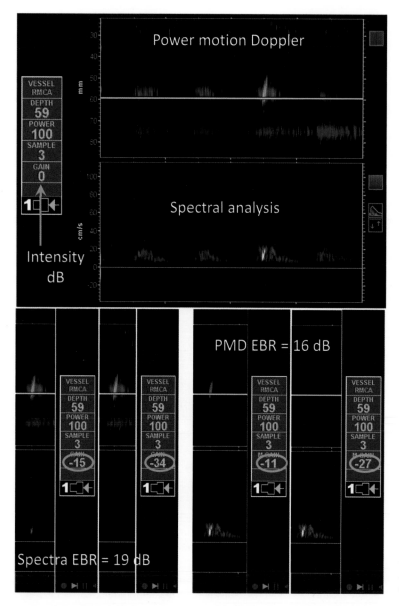

Figure 6.10 Embolic signals on power motion Doppler (PMD) and spectral TCD analyses. Measurements of signal intensity show how to determine embolus-to-blood (EBR) ratio for each modality by adjusting the gain to make the background blood flow disappear (flow intensity) and ES to disappear (maximum ES intensity). Intensity measurements are shown in orange ovals and derived EBR calculations are shown in respective PMD and spectral windows.

At our laboratory, we also measure the decrease in MFV if it occurs *during* breath holding or spontaneously when a nonaffected vessel shows the velocity increase in response to hypoventilation (Figure 6.13) [40]. If MFV decreases at the time of expected vasodilation, an intracranial steal is likely to be present. If this hemodynamic phenomenon is associated with concomitant neurological worsening, it represents the reversed Robin Hood syndrome. The **steal magnitude** (SM) correlates with degree of neurological worsening and is measured as follows [40]:

$$SM = (MFV_{min} - MFV_b / MFV_b) \times 100\%$$

where min is the minimum, or the lowest velocity during breath holding. More on this pattern and find-

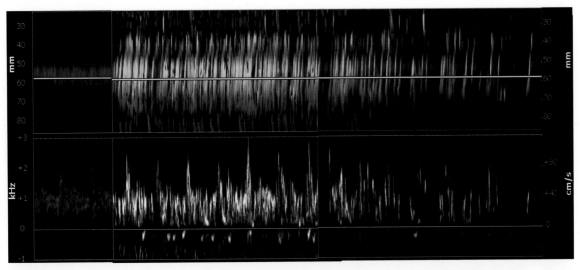

Figure 6.11 ES during right-to-left shunt testing with TCD and intravenous injection of 9 cc normal saline agitated with 1 cc room air. Interpretation: curtain ES appearance (International Consensus criteria) and Grade V+ (Spencer's logarithmic criteria) shunt gradings indicate one of the most functional right-to-left shunts present at rest.

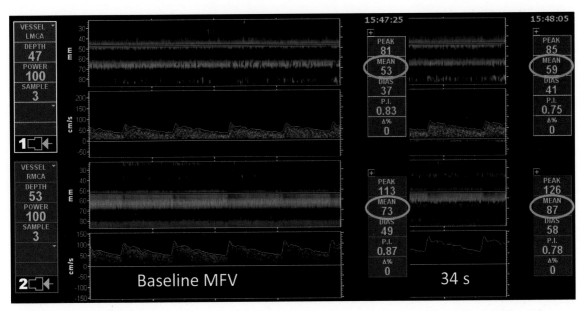

Figure 6.12 Bilateral TCD measurements of vasomotor reactivity (VMR) responses to voluntary 30-second breath holding in the MCAs. Breath-holding index (BHI) was calculated as follows: BHI LMCA = 0.38; BHI RMCA = 0.64. Interpretation: diminished VMR in the MCAs, left worse than right.

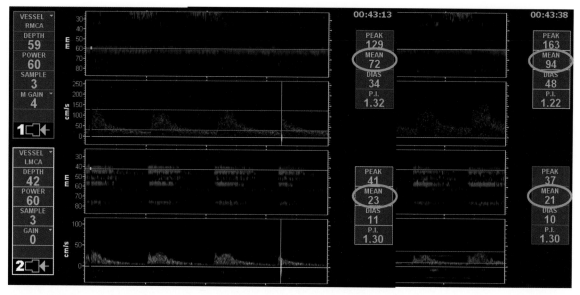

Figure 6.13 Bilateral VMR measurements in the MCAs showing intracranial blood flow steal due to CO_2 retention. VMR response is normal in the right MCA: Breath-holding index (BHI) RMCA = 1.02. Time corresponding velocity measurement in the LMCA shows paradoxical velocity decrease towards the end of voluntary breath holding (25 seconds) for BHI calculations. Therefore, the detected steal magnitude is: SM LMCA = –8.7%.

ings will be provided in other chapters. Steal can be observed during voluntary breath holding or other vasodilatory stimulation as well as spontaneously in patients with hypoventilation (e.g. obstructive sleep apnea, sleep disordered breathing, or obtunded poststroke) [40]. The steal can also be observed in the poststentotic arterial segments or arteries with the residual flow due to an acute occlusion (Figure 6.13). The next section explains how to semiquantitatively measure the abnormal waveforms detectable with intracranial occlusions.

As we are switching gears here, remember that there is still much to be learned from the waveforms. An **acute intracranial occlusion** is different from a chronic one because an *in situ* thrombus or an embolus often just partially obstructs the vessel, and the degree of obstruction can change over time. Some amount of detectable residual blood flow often exists around acute thromboembolic occlusions. Therefore, it can be identified through one of four **abnormal residual flow waveforms**, while recanalization is determined through improvement of the diastolic flow and subsequent appearance of the two waveforms that show normal or increased flow velocities. Together, these

waveforms represent the **Thrombolysis in Brain Ischemia (TIBI)** flow grading system (Figure 6.14) [41]:

1. absent,
2. minimal,
3. blunted,
4. dampened (or suppressed),
5. stenotic, and
6. normal.

In addition to the waveform analysis for the presence of an obstructive lesion, the velocity asymmetry can be calculated by comparison with a contralateral or nonaffected vessel [42, 43]. This asymmetry in general should be greater than 30% for homologous segments (that magnitude should account for differences in the angle of vessel intercept and breathing-mediated velocity fluctuations). Various asymmetry indexes have been proposed and validated in the literature, in addition to those in references [42] and [43]. The bottom line is: the greater the difference, the more convincing and predictive the findings appear. Any velocity asymmetry should be considered together with possible anatomic variability, as well as the presence or absence of flow diversion and collaterals.

Thrombolysis in brain ischemia (TIBI) waveforms

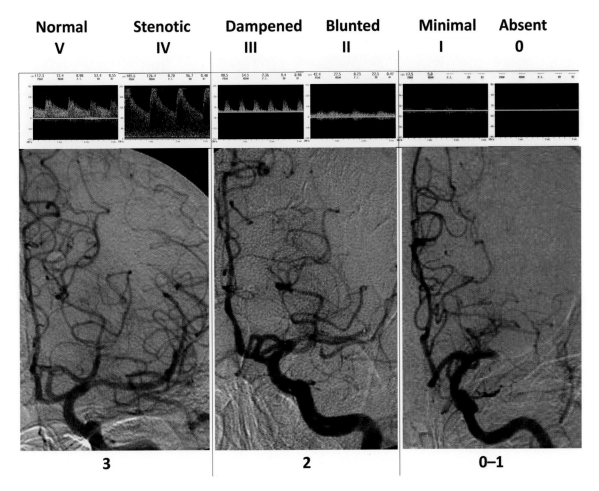

| Normal
V | Stenotic
IV | Dampened
III | Blunted
II | Minimal
I | Absent
0 |

Thrombolysis in myocardial infarction (TIMI) flow grades

Figure 6.14 Thrombolysis in Brain Ischemia (TIBI) flow grading system. This residual flow grading system was developed with the view to predict vessel appearance on cerebral angiography as graded by the Thrombolysis in Myocardial Infarction (TIMI) grades. The waveforms can be used to document the presence of a proximal arterial occlusion, focal recanalization, and estimate reperfusion of brain tissues.

Velocities are lower in the vessels like M2 MCA and TICA due to the angle of interception being closer to 90 degrees. In addition, the absence of flow diversion and a low resistance in the proximal feeding vessel help to avoid false-positive results. As a semiquantitative measurement system, the TIBI system with expanded definitions [44] is deployed in monitoring thrombolysis with TCD, determining recanalization, persistence of an occlusion, progression to a complete occlusion, or re-occlusion (Figure 6.15a).

Waveform patterns also play a very specific role in testing patients clinically suspect of being brain dead due to **cerebral circulatory arrest** [45]. If a positive diastolic flow is present in the M1 MCA or proximal

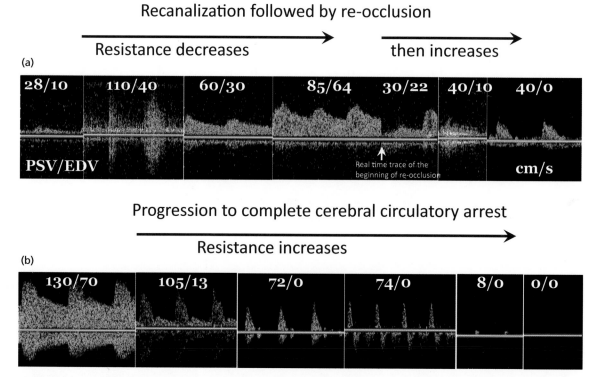

Figure 6.15 Changes in intracranial arterial waveforms with resistance increases due to progression of an occlusion in acute stroke and ICP changes. (**a**) Progression to a complete occlusion or re-occlusion. (**b**) Progression to a complete cerebral circulatory arrest (if confirmed also in contralateral MCA and basilar artery at stable BP values).

BA, this finding indicates no cerebral circulatory arrest at a given BP and ICP (Figure 6.15b). If the diastolic flow is absent, this may be found just prior to or after the arrest of the cerebral circulation. In these circumstances, measurements of BP (a must-to-know during any vascular examination) and ICP (if available) have to be done at the time of Doppler interrogation. Furthermore, measurements of PSV and trans-systolic time could be helpful because complete arrest is usually associated with lower PSV and very short trans-systolic times. The hallmark of cerebral circulatory arrest is the so-called **oscillating** or **reverberating** waveform (Figure 6.15b). This waveform simply demonstrates that the antegrade flow in systoli is replaced by a retrograde flow in diastoli. Even if some antegrade flow is sustained, it is not sufficient to maintain brain function in a brain without decompressed intracranial chamber, that is after the closure of fontanelles, and in the absence of any craniotomy. This finding points to a

grave prognosis. From hemodynamic stand-point, this waveform signifies that, at given BP values, as much blood is being pushed into the brain during systoli as is pushed back out in diastoli. There is no easy numeric way to document this flow pattern in a routine report, so we store the waveform as "a picture worth a thousand words" in this case, and mention the type of the waveform in the final report to support the comment of completeness of the arrest.

The knowledge and the ability to integrate all of the above TCD measures are important components of interpretation during real-time monitoring. If one sets out to monitor surgery, stenting, or acute stroke reperfusion, ultrasound can provide real-time measures of [46]:

1. hypoperfusion (Figure 6.16),
2. embolization (Figures 6.16 and 6.17),
3. thrombosis or re-occlusion (Figure 6.17),
4. hyperperfusion (Figure 6.17), and

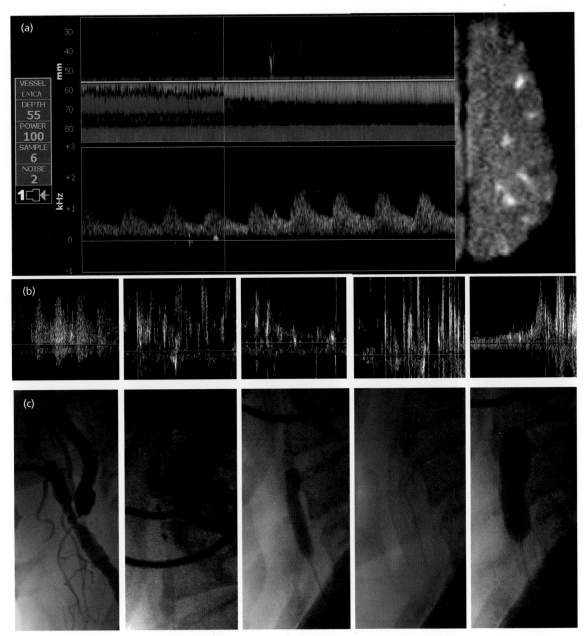

Figure 6.16 TCD findings of embolization and hypoperfusion. (**a**) Artery-to-artery embolization with corresponding recanalization changes during thrombolysis for a proximal ICA occlusion (MRI DWI sequence shows scattered cortical embolic ischemic lesions). (**b**) Frequent, mostly gaseous emboli during different stages of the ICA stenting procedure, commencement of hypoperfusion and subsequent reperfusion (middle and two right images) with stent deployment, and balloon inflation and deflation. Angiographic images (**c**) depict sequential stages of the carotid stenting procedure. From left to right: baseline angiographic findings, lesion crossing, initial balloon deployment, stent placement, and poststent-placement ballooning.

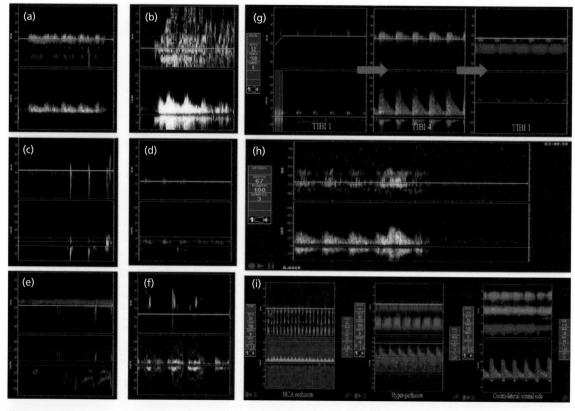

Figure 6.17 PMD TCD findings during intra-arterial (IA) catheter revascularization procedures in acute cerebral ischemia. (**a**) ES and velocity increase during contrast injection ("roadmap" creation at the beginning of the procedure). (**b**) ES and overall flow signal intensity increases during contrast injection during diagnostic angiographic "run". (**c**) ES with transient MFV decrease with Merci® retriever deployment. (**d**) Less intense ES and greater MFV decrease during Penumbra™ aspiration. (**e**) ES and MFV increase during intra-arterial tissue plasminogen activator injection. (**f**) High-intensity "halo-like" signals during catheter motion within the vessel with potentially harmful arterial flow disappearance during this catheter deployment/ re-positioning. (**g**) Prerevascularization TIBI grade 1 residual flow followed by evidence of partial recanalization after 1 hour (TIBI 3 flow appearance), and re-occlusion after next 40 minutes (TIBI 1 grade flow). (**h**) Air embolization of the MCA detected by a uniform increase in the flow intensity without catheter manipulation, corrected by repositioning of the sheath connector. (**i**) Hyperperfusion after stent deployment (1.5-times increase in the MFV compared with a homologous unaffected vessel).

5. procedure-specific changes such as flow reversal in the MCA with brain retroperfusion (Figure 6.18) [47, 48].

Several more measurements can be made during monitoring that aid predicting the development of a problem or ascertaining the mechanism of possible complication:

1. flow velocity reduction (% from baseline, diastolic abolishment), which at a constant angle of insonation is proportionate to the decrease in cerebral blood flow volume;

2. ES (massive numbers, occurrence during manipulations, or spontaneous) could point to the source of air or solid particle embolism;

3. flow reversal (change in flow direction with a stable angle of vessel intercept) in response to proximal vessel manipulations;

4. compensatory velocity and pulsatility changes or collateral flow recruitment (flow diversion, vasodilation, etc.);

5. hyperperfusion (flow velocity increase with pulsatility decrease);

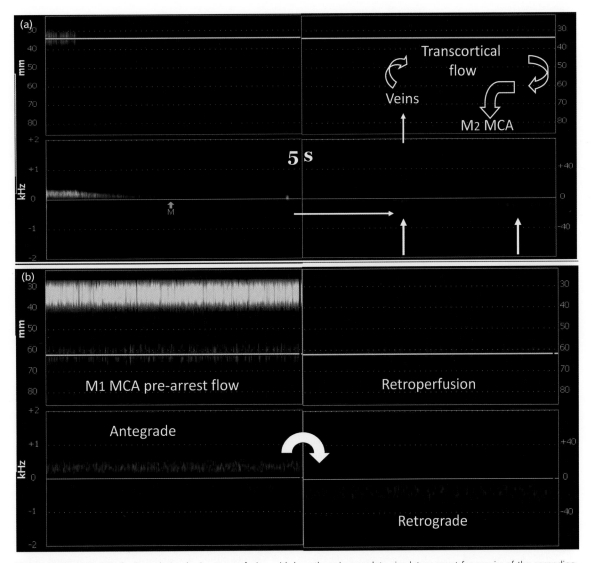

Figure 6.18 PMD TCD findings during brain retroperfusion with hypothermic complete circulatory arrest for repairs of the ascending aorta aneurysms. (**a**) An antegrade M2 MCA flow nonpulsatily bypass-induced signal prior to initiation of brain retroperfusion. Initiation of brain retroperfusion by blood infusion into the superior vena cava and M2 MCA flow reversal after 5 seconds of the bypass pump re-start. (**b**) Demonstration of the proximal M1–MCA flow reversal during brain retroperfusion.

6. thrombosis or re-occlusion (flow cessation, high-resistance patterns, etc.);

7. bilateral versus unilateral flow velocity, pulsatility, and waveform changes (for localization and differential diagnosis of systemic vs. local causes of blood flow changes).

This introduction to what ultrasound can measure is a very simplistic preview of what this technology can really offer at bedside. Returned echoes from blood flow, vessel walls, and parenchyma contain a wealth of information stored in the signal whether it is Doppler shift, intensity, amplitude, or other forms of energy transmission and signal conduction. Now, imagine that you can receive and process this information several thousand times a second. Yes, in one second you can have a myriad of measurements showing energy interaction with tissues that are conducting, absorbing, as well as transforming the signals. And this process can change any moment as endothelium function readjusts or reperfusion or flow depletion occur as well as vasomotor activity or drug actions commence. This is where the next frontier for ultrasound really is, and it would be a challenge to a new generation of scientists and clinicians, equipped with faster processing computer power and knowledge gained so far, to advance our understanding of vascular physiology, dynamic oxidative stress model, and tissue conditions under changing perfusion in real time.

Ultrasound offers a tool to measure or monitor a variety of tissue responses, and ways to deliver energy to target organs. The latter has already found its way into clinical practice through high-intensity focused ultrasound used to coagulate tissues while less intense energies offer positive biological effects suitable for sonothrombolysis, drug delivery, and action amplification. The next chapter will describe how to perform diagnostic ultrasound testing with currently available tools to obtain some of the measurements described in this chapter and to tailor testing to the particular patient presentation and neurological findings.

References

1. Alexandrov AV. *Cerebrovascular Ultrasound in Stroke Prevention and Treatment*, 2nd edn. Oxford: Wiley-Blackwell, 2011.
2. Valdueza JM, Shreiber SJ, Roehl JE, Klingebiel R. *Neurosonology and Neuroimaging of Stroke*. Stuttgart, Germany: Thieme, 2008.
3. Bartels E. *Color-Coded Duplex Ultrasonography of the Cerebral Arteries: Atlas and Manual*. Stuttgart, Germany: Schattauer, 1999.
4. Pellerito J, Polak J (eds). *Introduction to Vascular Ultrasonography*, 6th edn. Philadelphia: Saunders, 2012.
5. von Reutern GM, Budingen HJ. *Ultrasound Diagnosis of Cerebrovascular Disease*. Stuttgart: Georg Thieme Verlag, 1993.
6. Polak JF, Pencina MJ, Pencina KM, *et al*. Carotid-wall intima-media thickness and cardiovascular events. *N Engl J Med* 2011; **365**: 213–21.
7. Pourcelot L, Tranquart F, De Bray JM, *et al*. Ultrasound characterization and quantification of carotid atherosclerosis lesions (Review). *Minerva Cardioangiol* 1999; **47**: 15–24.
8. Polak JF, Shemanski L, O'Leary DH, *et al*. Hypoechoic plaque at US of the carotid artery: an independent risk factor for incident stroke in adults aged 65 years or older. Cardiovascular Health Study. *Radiology* 1998; **208**: 649–54.
9. Bluth EI, Sunshine JH, Lyons JB, *et al*. Power Doppler imaging: initial evaluation as a screening examination for carotid artery stenosis. *Radiology* 2000; **215**: 791–800.
10. Gosling RG, King DH. Arterial assessment by Doppler-shift ultrasound. *Proc Roy Soc Med* 1974; **67**: 447–9.
11. Pourcellot L. *Applications Cliniques de l'Examen Doppler Transcutane. Les Colloques de l'Institute National de la Sante et de la Recherche Medicale*. INSERM, 1974, pp. 213–40.
12. Blackshear WM, Phillips DJ, Chikos PM, *et al*. Carotid artery velocity patterns in normal and stenotic vessels. *Stroke* 1980; **11**: 67–71.
13. Grant EG, Benson CB, Moneta GL, *et al*. Carotid artery stenosis: gray-scale and Doppler US diagnosis – Society of Radiologists in Ultrasound Consensus Conference. *Radiology* 2003; **229**: 340–6.
14. Spencer MP, Reid JM. Quantitation of carotid stenosis with continuous wave Doppler ultrasound. *Stroke* 1979; **10**: 326–30.
15. Alexandrov AV, Sloan MA, Wong LKS, *et al*. Practice standards for transcranial Doppler (TCD) ultrasound. Part I. Test performance. *J Neuroimaging* 2007; **17**: 11–18.
16. Alexandrov AV, Sloan MA, Tegeler CH, *et al*; for the American Society of Neuroimaging Practice Guidelines Committee. Practice standards for transcranial Doppler (TCD) ultrasound. Part II. Clinical indications and expected outcomes. *J Neuroimaging* 2012; **22**: 215–24.
17. Michel E, Zernikow B. Gosling's pulsatility index revisited. *Ultrasound Med Biol* 1998; **24**: 597–9.
18. Alexandrov AV. Extra- and intracranial waveform analysis algorithm, descriptions, classifications and differential diagnosis. *J Vasc Ultrasound* 2012; **36**: 103–12.
19. Lindegaard KF, Nornes H, Bakke SJ, *et al*. Cerebral vasospasm after subarachnoid haemorrhage investigated by means of transcranial Doppler ultrasound. *Acta Neurochir* (Wien) 1988; **42** (Suppl.): P81–4.
20. Soustiel JF, Shik V, Shreiber R, *et al*. Basilar vasospasm diagnosis: investigation of a modified "Lindegaard Index" based on imaging studies and blood velocity measurements of the basilar artery. *Stroke* 2002; **33**: 72–7.
21. Sviri GE, Lewis DH, Correa R, *et al*. Basilar artery vasospasm and delayed posterior circulation ischemia after aneurysmal subarachnoid hemorrhage. *Stroke* 2004; **35**: 1867–72.

22. Sviri GE, Ghodke B, Britz GW, et al. Transcranial Doppler grading criteria for basilar artery vasospasm. *Neurosurgery* 2006; **59**: 360–6.

23. Spencer MP, Campbell SD, Sealey JL, et al. Experiments on decompression bubbles in the circulation using ultrasonic and electromagnetic flowmeters. *J Occup Med* 1969; **11**: 238–44.

24. Padayachee TS, Gosling RG, Bishop CC, et al. Transcranial measurement of blood velocities in the basal cerebral arteries using pulsed Doppler ultrasound: a method of assessing the Circle of Willis. *Ultrasound Med Biol* 1986; **12**: 5–14.

25. Deverall PB, Padayachee TS, Parsons S, et al. Ultrasound detection of micro-emboli in the middle cerebral artery during cardiopulmonary bypass surgery. *Eur J Cardiothorac Surg* 1988; **2**: 256–60.

26. Spencer MP, Thomas GI, Nicholls SC, Sauvage LR. Detection of middle cerebral artery emboli during carotid endarterectomy using transcranial Doppler ultrasonography. *Stroke* 1990; **21**: 415–23.

27. Russell D. The detection of cerebral emboli using Doppler ultrasound. In: Newell DW, Aaslid R (eds), *Transcranial Doppler*. New York: Raven Press, 1992: pp. 52–8.

28. The International Cerebral Hemodynamics Society Consensus Statement. *Stroke* 1995; **26**: 1123.

29. Moehring MA, Spencer MP. Power M-mode Doppler (PMD) for observing cerebral blood flow and tracking emboli. *Ultrasound Med Biol* 2002; **28**: 49–57.

30. Tong DC, Bolger A, Albers GW. Incidence of transcranial Doppler-detected cerebral microemboli in patients referred for echocardiography. *Stroke* 1994; **25**: 2138–41.

31. Georgiadis D, Grosset DG, Kelman A, et al. Prevalence and characteristics of intracranial microemboli signals in patients with different types of prosthetic cardiac valves. *Stroke* 1994; **25**: 587–92.

32. Lao AY, Sharma VK, Tsivgoulis G, et al. Detection of right-to-left shunts: Comparison between the International Consensus and Spencer Logarithmic Scale Criteria. *J Neuroimaging* 2008; **18**: 402–6.

33. Ackerstaff RG, Jansen C, Moll FL, et al. The significance of microemboli detection by means of transcranial Doppler ultrasonography monitoring in carotid endarterectomy. *J Vasc Surg* 1995; **21**: 963–9.

34. Spencer MP, Moehring MA, Jesurum J et al. Power m-mode transcranial Doppler for diagnosis of patent foramen ovale and assessing transcatheter closure. *J Neuroimaging* 2004; **14**: 342–9.

35. Silverstrini M, Vernieri F, Pasqualetti P, et al. Impaired vasomotor reactivity and risk of stroke in patients with asymptomatic carotid artery stenosis. *JAMA* 2000; **283**: 2122–7.

36. Palazzo P, Balucani C, Barlinn K, et al. Association of reversed Robin Hood syndrome with risk of stroke recurrence. *Neurology* 2010; **75**: 2003–8.

37. Ringelstein EB, Van Eyck S, Mertens I. Evaluation of cerebral vasomotor reactivity by various vasodilating stimuli: comparison of CO_2 to acetazolamide. *J Cereb Blood Flow Metab* 1992; **12**: 162–8.

38. Schreiber SJ, Gottschalk S, Weih M, et al. Assessment of blood flow velocity and diameter of the middle cerebral artery during the acetazolamide provocation test by use of transcranial Doppler sonography and MR imaging. *AJNR Am J Neuroradiol* 2000; **21**: 1207–11.

39. Markus HS, Harrison MJ. Estimation of cerebrovascular reactivity using transcranial Doppler, including the use of breath-holding as the vasodilatory stimulus. *Stroke* 1992; **23**: 668–73.

40. Alexandrov AV, Sharma VK, Lao AY, et al. Reversed Robin Hood syndrome in acute ischemic stroke patients. *Stroke* 2007; **38**: 3045–8.

41. Demchuk AM, Burgin WS, Christou I, et al. Thrombolysis in Brain Ischemia (TIBI) transcranial Doppler flow grades predict clinical severity, early recovery, and mortality in patients treated with tissue plasminogen activator. *Stroke* 2001; **32**: 89–93.

42. Zanette EM, Fieschi C, Bozzao L, et al. Comparison of cerebral angiography and transcranial Doppler sonography in acute stroke. *Stroke* 1989; **20**: 899–03.

43. Saqqur M, Hill MD, Alexandrov AV, et al. Derivation of power M-Mode transcranial Doppler criteria for angiographic proven MCA occlusion. *J Neuroimaging* 2006; **16**: 323–8.

44. Alexandrov AV. Ultrasound-enhanced thrombolysis for stroke: clinical significance. *Eur J Ultrasound* 2002; **16**: 131–40.

45. Ducrocq X, Hassler W, Moritake K, et al. Consensus opinion on diagnosis of cerebral circulatory arrest using Doppler-sonography: Task Force Group on cerebral death of the Neurosonology Research Group of the World Federation of Neurology. *J Neurol Sci* 1998; **159**: 145–50.

46. Spencer MP. Transcranial Doppler monitoring and causes of stroke from carotid endarterectomy. *Stroke* 1997; **28**: 685–91.

47. Sakahashi H, Hashimoto A, Aomi S, et al. Transcranial Doppler measurement of middle cerebral artery blood flow during continuous retrograde cerebral perfusion. *Nippon Kyobu Geka Gakkai Zasshi* 1994; **42**: 1851–7 (Japanese).

48. Razumovsky AY, Tseng EE, Hanley DF, Baumgartner WA. Cerebral hemodynamic changes during retrograde brain perfusion in dogs. *J Neuroimaging* 2001; **11**: 171–8.

"Do not fight with the probe – probe always wins"
Sonographers advice for hand-held examinations

Approaching the patient and neurological considerations

Once cerebral ischemia has produced neurological symptoms, the cause may only be transiently present in the vasculature. Thus, the vascular assessment is often performed as if "looking for a smoking gun" after one has heard a shot. Delaying assessment decreases the chances of detecting the source of a problem. Furthermore, structural and snap-shot type vascular imaging may not provide all the needed answers. In this setting, ultrasound is a handy tool to be deployed with the aim of linking the neurological dysfunction to the malperfusion culprit in real time. Ultrasound offers the convenience of bedside, real-time assessment of physiological as well as morphological information, and is complimentary to the physical examination and other imaging tests.

The neurological examination can localize the lesion within the nervous system, and these skills are taught throughout physician training. For health professionals caring for stroke patients, focused and structured neurological examination skills can be acquired through learning the National Institutes of Health Stroke Scale (NIHSS) [1], included in Chapter 1. Although the NIHSS measures stroke severity, findings of the neurological examination are not specific as to the level of an arterial obstruction nor to its type (i.e. embolism, thrombosis, hypoperfusion, etc.), which could have been the cause of the brain dysfunc-tion. Furthermore, in patients with resolved deficits the neurological findings are normal and clinicians have to reconstruct symptoms and signs from patients' or by-standers' recollections.

Like a stethoscope, ultrasound provides a tool to examine the precerebral and intracranial vessels, thus expanding the physical examination. I use ultrasound as an extension of my neurological assessment, making it a **neurovascular examination**. This combined neurovascular assessment (in an abbreviated form tailored to a specific patient's presentation) can be repeated rapidly and as needed if the condition of a patient changes or when a therapy is administered.

If one has the luxury of time, a complete neurovascular examination can help to avoid false-negative or false-positive results, and it could offer even more clues. The details of the neurological examination and differential diagnosis are covered by many well-respected textbooks. The same is true about ultrasound. After finishing the detailed neurological examination, a physician may order a complete carotid and TCD examination, which may take some time to complete and interpret. These tests, if done meticulously in a laboratory that carries out self-validation studies as required by accreditation processes, can yield good-to-excellent agreement with angiography [2–5]. Moreover, these tests themselves can take up to 1 hour or more to complete, depending on the case complexity, sonographer skills, and the need for additional specific TCD examinations, such as vasomotor reactivity, shunt and emboli detection, etc. And again, the complete scanning protocols are available elsewhere and are taught to sonographers during their training (complete extra- and intracranial scanning

---

Neurovascular Examination: The Rapid Evaluation of Stroke Patients Using Ultrasound Waveform Interpretation, First Edition.
Andrei V. Alexandrov.
© 2013 Andrei V. Alexandrov. Published 2013 by Blackwell Publishing Ltd.

protocols can be found in *Cerebrovascular Ultrasound in Stroke Prevention and Treatment* [6] or elsewhere in the standard vascular ultrasound textbooks [7–10]).

As of the beginning of this millennium, clinicians routinely order carotid ultrasound, fewer do so for TCD, and very few have mastered the skills to perform all available neurovascular ultrasound tests themselves. Part of the reason for this is the complexity of ultrasound testing, part is the lack of understanding of what ultrasound can offer, and part is a minimalistic approach to stroke diagnostic workup and care. Further problems arise if the neurological training is focused mainly on the first two "Ws", **Where?** and **What?**, as opposed to the third, **Why?** The last one is the subject of particular interest here as stroke pathogenic mechanisms link the first two Ws together, and provide clues for how to treat or prevent this condition. With the mind set for a fast and curative approach to stroke, clinicians need to find answers in a speedy manner. Our stroke care philosophy is: "find reasons to treat", act fast, tailor treatment to the specific stroke mechanism, have a plan to prevent complications, and efficiently respond to changing conditions.

The question is how to combine both the neurological assessment and vascular ultrasound testing so that at rounds or in an emergency at the bedside one can observe or elicit the most informative signs and gain most insights from the initial neurological and vascular findings – and obtain this information "on a dime," that is with sparse initial clinical information and a few waveforms or images obtainable in the emergency setting. Our assessments should be fast, that is it should not delay the door-to-treatment time in acute stroke beyond a few unavoidable processes required by the usual standard of care.

One should spend enough time to learn the neurological examination, diagnosis, and differential diagnosis of cerebrovascular diseases, and master the complete carotid and TCD scanning protocols, before embarking on an "observe-and-test-only-what-is-important" practice of an abbreviated emergent assessment at bedside. Future progress in the development of faster, less operator-dependent, and more portable ultrasound scanners will one day make a complete and quick neurovascular examination a reality for many clinicians.

In this chapter, I will use an acute cerebral ischemia as an example of a situation where a complete neurological examination and complete carotid duplex and TCD tests are impractical due to limits posed by a decreasing benefit from reperfusion therapies over time from symptom onset. Evaluation of an acute stroke patient leaves no room for "twiddling your thumbs" or performing long or unnecessary tests. Instead, clinicians must use the high-yield assessments that are rapid and deliver information relevant to subsequent management decisions. As we joke on service, one will automatically fail the stroke rotation if, in the presence of an obvious and disabling neurological deficit, the Babinski's reflex is elicited before administration of the tissue plasminogen activator (tPA) bolus.

Suppose a patient presents with anterior circulation symptoms such as gaze deviation and inattention, signs that are easily observed and quickly tested. Starting the vascular part of the examination with the anterior circulation will likely have the highest yield. When pressed for time, I start with the *intracranial* ultrasound examination because the offending thrombus, if any, or its extension causing hypoperfusion, is most likely to be found intracranially at the level of the circle of Willis or its proximal branches. When time permits, I start on the nonaffected side to see how the presumably normal or nonaffected vessels look like for subsequent comparison with the affected side. If even more time is available, knowing what is going on in the neck can help interpret intracranial findings. I will therefore cover the extracranial vessel examination first, as mastering this part is critical for subsequent understanding of intracranial findings and differential diagnosis.

Extracranial vessel examination

The extracranial duplex examination starts with a quick transverse B-mode sweep from the CCA to the jaw level on the symptomatic brain side. Position the transducer at the midcervical level in front of the sternocleidomastoid muscle, and adjust it medially or laterally to place the round-shaped CCA in the middle of the image (Figure 7.1). Adjust the depth of scanning accordingly. If confused with the jugular vein, gently apply pressure and the vein will decrease in size immediately (it will become triangular shaped or collapse, so apply very gentle pressure!) while the CCA

B-mode surveillance ## Pathology on power + B-mode

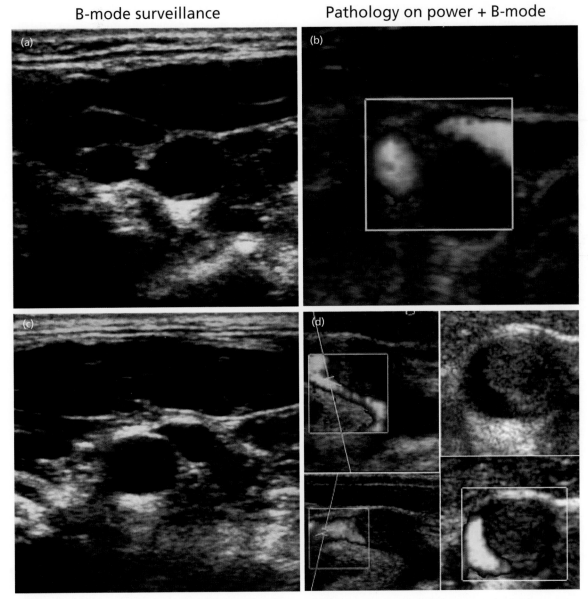

Figure 7.1 Initial surveillance steps of the extracranial vasculature. (**a, c**) Likely patent CCA and ICA/ECA. (**b, d**) Abnormalities revealed by B-mode: absent flow in the ICA due to distal occlusion (**b**) and an intraluminal thrombus in the ICA (**d**).

will remain round in shape. Scan up and down the artery barrel. This basically tells me if:

1. any plaque or intraluminal thrombus or flap is seen (Figure 7.1), and

2. if all three (CCA, ICA, and ECA) vessels can be visualized proximal to the level of the jaw.

I then add power mode or color flow to see if (Figure 7.1):

1. flow in one of the carotid bifurcation vessels is missing (with or without plaque or intraluminal thrombus),

2. one or both have a high-resistance appearance,

3. the detectable flow in the residual lumen reduction matches plaque protrusion, or

4. all three (CCA, ICA, and ECA) appear normal, and

5. subsequent appearance of the vessels in a longitudinal view (both B-mode and power or color flow) matches the above findings (Figure 7.1).

I will examine in turn the points above because it literally takes less than 30 seconds to check for all of the above and have some clues from the "get-go" as to what you might be dealing with, that is proximal ICA involvement, distal lesion, etc.

Remember, a "missing" (or "not found", i.e. not visualized) vessel does not mean it is occluded. Failure to see a normal carotid bifurcation means either: (a) it is too high (i.e. above the jaw), (b) one of the vessels takes off at a really unfavorable angle (less common in power mode plus transverse visualization), or (c) there is no flow in one of the vessels (an artifact vs. occlusion).

If flow in one vessel appears to be missing, I first check the machine settings to make sure that sluggish or high-resistance flow can be properly displayed (gain, box angulation, velocity scale). Remember the rule that if something is wrong or does not make sense during ultrasound examination, the likely causes should be considered as follows:

1. a technical error (often the best first answer or first issue to rule out);

2. anatomy and systemic hemodynamic reasons (almost always at play to some extent);

and only then

3. relevant cerebrovascular pathology.

Therefore, I look again at optimized B-mode/ flow images to confirm that the presumed-missing vessel could be identified below the level of the jaw, and that lack of flow is not a function of an unfavorable angle or due to high resistance (like the ECA appearance at the end of cardiac cycle), or the bulb being too large. In the latter case, the flow velocity in the bulb may be too slow to be readily depicted by color or power imaging.

Then, I check if the vessel is patent at this level or there are any intraluminal echoes that would be consistent with either a pre-existing plaque, new thrombus (Figure 7.1), or an intimal tear (flap). Remember that calcium in a plaque can produce shadowing and obscure the luminal flow. In this case, some flow distal to the shadow will be seen. Flaps can be an artifact produced by a bright reflector between the transducer and the common or internal carotid arteries (Figure 7.2).

If the vessel has no intraluminal echoes on B-mode, I expect to see either no flow or a high-resistance flow pattern with absent diastolic flow, findings that imply the presence of a complete occlusion distal to the site of insonation. In this case, both ECA and ICA will appear on power mode as intermittently flashing (analogous with a yellow traffic light). Remember that under normal conditions and with proper flow scale settings, ICA is constantly present through the systoli and diastoli whereas ECA is "flashing," mostly during systoli.

If intraluminal echoes are present, I would like to see if the residual lumen appearance on power mode matches that of a structural lesion on B-mode (Figure 7.1d images). This is particularly useful if some degree of an atheromatous stenosis, or intraluminal thrombus, or a proximal dissection is suspected. If a newly discovered plaque is small and little flow is visualized on power mode, check the settings and suspect a distal lesion when a high-resistance flow is truly present.

If a normal vessel appearance is noted extracranially (i.e. CCA is filling with power mode signal throughout its stem, and its bifurcation has vessels with low- and high-resistance patterns), it is reassuring (Figures 7.3 and 7.4). If time permits, I reconfirm vessel identification on color flow by visualizing ECA branches and on spectral Doppler waveforms with tapping the temporal artery (Figure 7.4). However, both ICA and ECA appearances can be misleading in patients with suspected atherothrombotic or embolic carotid occlusions, Horner's syndrome, neck pain, or even in patients with mild or resolved stroke symptoms. Note that ICA can become externalized (i.e. show flow patterns of high resistance), and ECA can internalize [11], that is that of low-resistance pattern (Figure 7.5). A unilateral ophthalmic artery reversal is the reason for the diastolic velocity increase relative to peak systoli in the ECA, and the distal lesion in the ICA is often the cause of ICA diastolic velocity decrease and sharpening of its waveform.

If the normal patterns are seen in the neck, I simply make a note if the ICA has any plaque at origin (Figure 7.3). I then question if the ICA, its distal and terminal segments, or main branches are still patent distal to

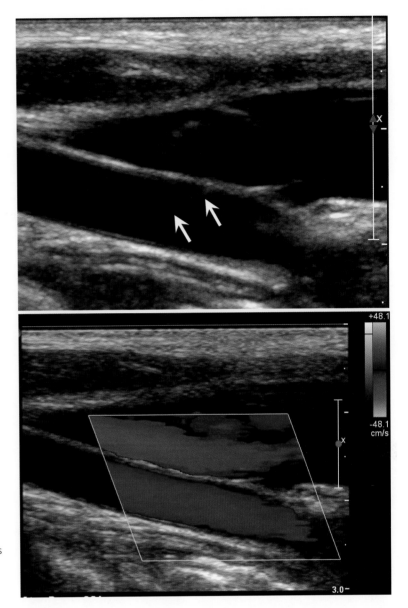

Figure 7.2 An artifact on B-mode suggesting an intimal flap in the CCA. Note a bright reflector such as the near wall of the jugular vein that produces this artifact. Color flow application rules out the presence of a false lumen above the artifactual lining on B-mode.

the site of insonation. Remember, an acute lesion could cause partial obstruction, and vessel patency may change over time. More information will be derived from the spectral Doppler.

After a brief longitudinal examination with B-mode, power, or color flow, spectral analysis can be the judge of lesion severity or point to its location if it was not directly visualized by the above mentioned modalities. The mid-CCA waveforms are quick to obtain (Figure

7.3). I rock the transducer to switch from CCA appearance parallel to the transducer/ skin surface interface to the one "at an angle," depending on where I am going to sample spectral waveforms. This helps to put a preset, oblique color flow box to the right or left of the image, and to proceed faster with a preset 60-degree angle-corrected spectral Doppler interrogation. To save time, I try to place the flow divider to the left of the image and sample mid-to-distal CCA to

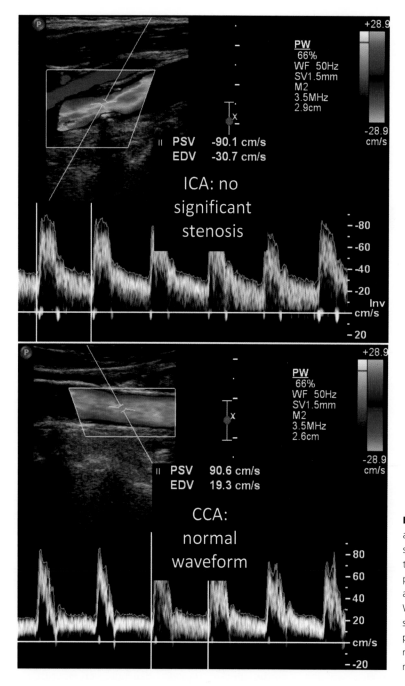

PW
66%
WF 50Hz
SV1.5mm
M2
3.5MHz
2.9cm

PSV   -90.1 cm/s
EDV   -30.7 cm/s

ICA: no significant stenosis

PW
66%
WF 50Hz
SV1.5mm
M2
3.5MHz
2.6cm

PSV   90.6 cm/s
EDV   19.3 cm/s

CCA: normal waveform

Figure 7.3 Color flow guided brief assessment of the CCA and ICA flow/ spectral waveforms. Rock the transducer to place the vessels of interest along the preset color flow/ spectral Doppler angulations of 60 degrees to save time. Waveforms and velocities are typical of no significant obstruction to flow in the precerebral vasculature. Note a small nonstenosing plaque at the ICA bulb with no significant velocity elevation.

the far right of the image (a maneuver described in Chapter 6). In addition to seeing CCA waveform unaffected by its distal dilation/ bifurcation, I also obtain peak systolic velocity measurement here as the denominator of the ICA/CCA PSV ratio.

If the CCA peak systolic velocity is within normal limits in an adult patient (i.e. usually 50 cm/s or more) and there is a reasonable diastolic flow (i.e. more than 15 cm/s) (Figure 7.3), I'm more assured that I'm not missing a severe ICA obstruction. If the diastolic flow

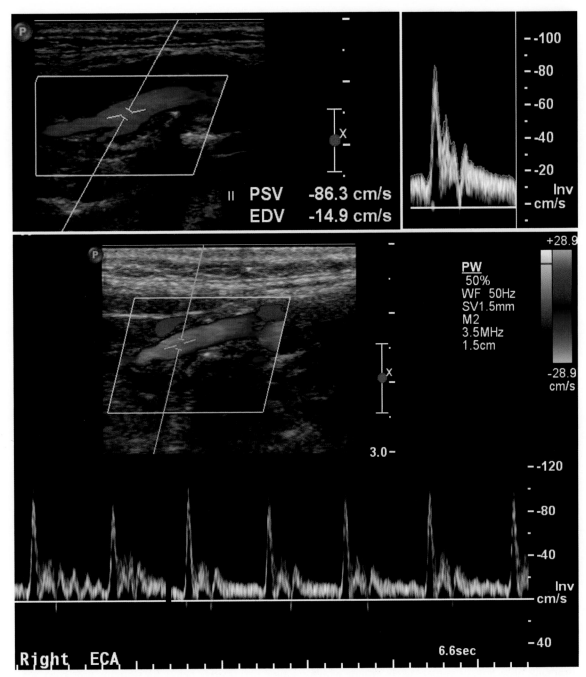

Figure 7.4 Typical appearance of the ECA. A branch is seen on color flow, spectral waveform shows a high-resistance pattern and it responds to the temporal artery tapping.

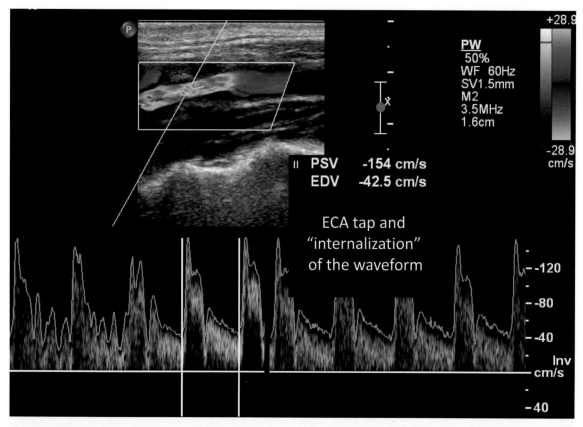

Figure 7.5 Internalization of the ECA in a case of a chronic ICA occlusion. Note the response to the temporal artery tap.

is low or absent, or the peak systolic velocity is decreased and CCA waveforms appear high resistant or suppressed, I check the spectral Doppler scale and filter settings and suspect a significant lesion in the ICA. By advancing the scanning field to the bifurcation level, I would like to capture the plaque presence (if any), match the residual lumen appearance with the structure of a lesion, and to perform a quick spectral Doppler interrogation to decide if the lesion is less than 50% (Figure 7.3), ≥50%, near-occlusive, or completely occlusive. The B-mode appearance will again be helpful to decide if the lesion is a plaque, thrombus, dissection, or you are likely dealing with a distal lesion.

If the ICA is difficult to visualize due to high carotid bifurcation, I ask (or help) the patient to slightly turn their head away from the examination side and raise their chin slightly up while I'm moving the transducer into a more posterior approach behind the angle of

the jaw. If this does not suffice, I turn the transducer from longitudinal (i.e. parallel to the sternocleidomastoid muscle aiming straight downwards) to a more oblique approach aiming more cephalad. This may jeopardize the angle for Doppler interrogation but may in turn visualize the vessel lumen and flow in power mode.

If the carotid surveillance yields normal results, have a quick look at the unilateral vertebral artery. There may be surprises. If the patient's symptoms are from the posterior circulation, consider starting with the vertebral artery (VA) assessment on the neck, if time permits (see below for scanning protocols).

The VA in the neck is found by switching slightly laterally and posteriorly from the longitudinal view of the CCA to visualize the transverse processes (shadows), and by placing power or color flow imaging to detect any flow in between those shadows (Figure 7.6). If the VA is not found, remember, it does not

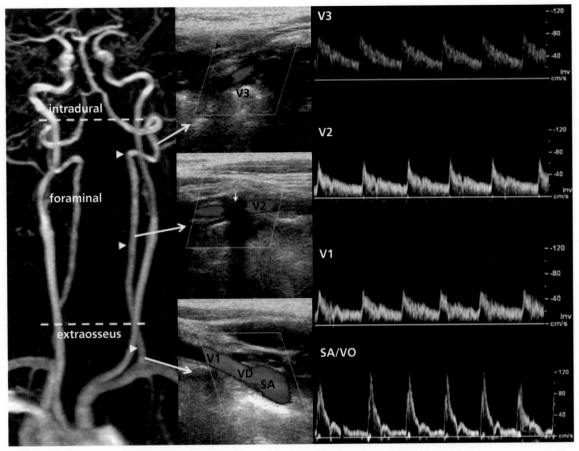

Figure 7.6 Extracranial examination of the vertebral artery segments. Note the segmental nature of the VA flow assessment and the waveform/ velocity changes from its origin to the midcervical segment.

mean it is acutely occluded. I quickly add a larger sample Doppler gate (3–5 mm) and place it along the structural image that is most convincing of the VA interception. I always keep gain levels high enough to see some noise on spectral display – this is assurance not to miss very weak flow signals. I expand this interrogation proximally to the origin and distally following the VA course in between the processes or outside the bony canal. To visualize the VA origin, I sometimes have to ask the patient to reach with their hand as close as possible to their knee on the side of the examination. This maneuver tilts the clavicle down, and opens just enough scanning access to move along the VA course to its origin. Remember, the vertebral arteries have an impressive ability to collateralize and reconstitute distally to a lesion, thus making diagnosis

more difficult. Obstructed segments can be covered by transverse processes or lesions could be multiple and variable in length.

Intracranial vessel examination

This section is applicable to both transcranial duplex imaging and transcranial Doppler examination, with or without contrast agents, tests that can be used in emergency situations at the bedside. Images can be convincing ("seeing is believing"), suggestive, misleading, or erroneous. While clinicians are enamored with fast-evolving structural imaging to locate the problem, future progress in this area should improve our understanding of how brain vessels continue to function in real time to compensate for these lesions or when they yield to the disease. Our treatments should evolve from a "one shot for all" approach to highly efficient and tailor-made real-time interventions. Ultrasound can provide information to adapt to, or proactively change, hemodynamic conditions induced by multiple factors, among which proximal reperfusion or re-occlusion are directly assessable by ultrasound. Ultrasound findings can reveal, in real time, perfusion changes, with blood levels of carbon dioxide, cardiac output, endothelial function, etc. Our tools to evaluate brain vessels and microcirculation should also improve to match the progress of imaging brain parenchyma. But I digressed, again.

One should know the advantages and limitations of each scanning method prior to choosing one and making quick decisions from test results. This becomes particularly important when one has to identify an intracranial arterial lesion, if any, in the shortest time possible. Like with extracranial scanning, you should learn intracranial scanning techniques and practice complete examinations before you embark on emergent and abbreviated assessments.

If time is available (by that I mean standard of care activities other than ultrasound still leave some time before reperfusion therapy is initiated, or treatment has already started), obtain information about normal vessel location and waveforms as a reference. This usually can be found in a segment on the nonaffected side that is homologous to the one under suspicion from the neurological symptoms. This also helps to establish the presence of a window for insonation and may give immediate clues to pathophysiological hemodynamic changes, that is compensatory contralateral velocity increase with collaterals to compensate for hemodynamically significant carotid or vertebrobasilar obstructions.

If pressed for time, start with the transtemporal window on the affected side because the anterior circulation is most often affected by stroke. Aim slightly upwards and anterior from the transducer position just above and in front of the ear canal, that is the midtemporal window. With imaging, make sure that you visualize the following (Figure 7.7):
1. darker area of the unilateral temporal lobe;
2. the third ventricle reflections (depth 7–8 cm);
3. contralateral skull (scanning depth about 15 cm in adults).

After these B-mode landmarks are found, apply color or power mode for flow assessment (more details of complete transcranial duplex scanning protocols can be found elsewhere [7, 8]). Make sure that the size of the box in not excessive to the task, that is extending to the contralateral vessels that would be beyond the scope of necessary investigation. Once the box is placed, look at the following (Figure 7.7):
1. any flow in the MCA main stem (usually at depth 40–60 mm) or branches (30–40 mm);
2. any flow in the terminal ICA (usually a round spot at 60–70 mm);
3. any flow in the ACA (usually away from the probe at 60–80 mm); and
4. any flow in the PCA or PCommA (probe angulation may need to be adjusted as well as the size of the flow imaging box).

Do not forget that a branch may be obstructed and the appearance of the rest may be normal on the flow image. Remember to "go with the flow" and open/visualize vessels as shallow or as deep as possible to look at all vessels that are expected to be found at the above-noted ranges. Good-quality flow imaging surveillance provides the basis for Doppler spectral interrogation (Figure 7.8). Spectral Doppler waveforms should be documented to support the diagnosis of the vessel patency, proximal occlusion, distal occlusion, or tandem lesions.

Whether you start with learning duplex or TCD scanning techniques, remember to always check for the following at the beginning of the examination:
1. full power setting when starting transtemporal examination;
2. large sample volume (≥10 mm) for a single channel TCD or 3-mm sample volume for power motion Doppler (PMD) TCD;
3. initial application of the transducer over midtemporal window with slightly upwards and anterior angulation (targeting the anterior circulation/ diencephalic plane);
4. steady transducer positioning with slow small circular movements around the midtemporal window to get returned echoes if the initial application did not yield the window for insonation right away;
5. reapply gel and patiently restart scanning with more pressure on the transducer to achieve better probe–skin interface if the initial attempts failed to locate any flow signals;

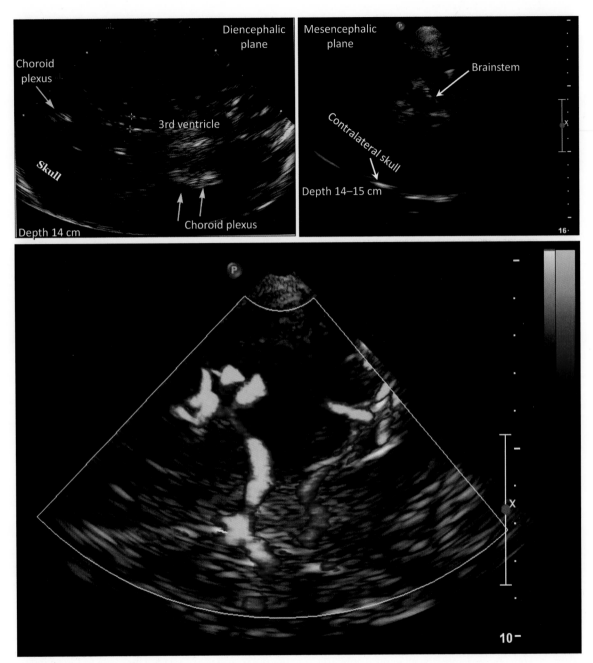

Figure 7.7 Typical B-mode findings during the initial steps of intracranial duplex examination. Anatomic landmarks as well as the depth and spatial course of the vessels aid rapid vessel identification and help guide Doppler interrogation.

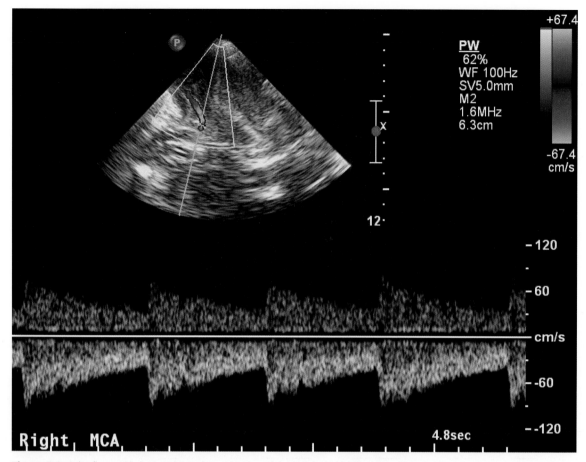

Figure 7.8 Color flow guided spectral Doppler assessment of the terminal ICA bifurcation. Note that the signal above the baseline has a velocity slightly less than the signal below the baseline, which is not pathological. This is due to a less-optimal angle of interception of the terminal ICA opening into the MCA (towards the probe) compared to the ACA origin (away from the probe). This site of spectral interrogation has one of the highest yields when searching for a proximal anterior circulation occlusion.

6. reangulate the transducer posteriorly over the midtemporal window to see if posterior circulation vessels can be detected from the same window (this is often helpful with the proximal MCA or TICA occlusions to differentiate no window vs. no flow);

7. learn to track flow signals from normal vessels to obstructed ones by remembering anatomic landmarks, transducer angualtions to intercept certain vessels in relation to these landmarks, and by steady aiming at signals with decreasing velocities/ intensities proximal to the depths with no detectable pulsations.

Incomplete examination is the most common source of error, particularly when done in a rush. Although most stroke-causing lesions are found in the MCA, other vessels can also be affected or their waveforms can provide clues to unmask a distal MCA lesion (i.e. flow diversion to ACA or PCA with an M2 MCA occlusion). Finding collaterals implies the presence of an arterial obstruction proximal to the collateral channel, and could help detect tandem lesions such as involving the ICA and MCA [12, 13].

In patients with resolved symptoms, pure motor or sensory deficits or with uncertain localization, I start examination with the anterior circulation vessels. However, I also expand it to the posterior circulation vessels to make sure that this less-frequently affected but still significant circulatory bed is examined. Every clinician should be prepared to stumble upon a vertebrobasilar stroke presentation, which could be most confusing.

Emergent neurovascular assessment

Upon approaching the patient for the first time, I briefly observe the initial patient behavior or responses, if any (I'm often present when paramedics bring the patient in and together with nurses we move the patient from the ambulance stretcher to the ER bed or to the CT scanner). While listening to a brief report given to ER personnel or by them to me, I quickly look for an obvious and disabling deficit (e.g. the patient looks away from the side that is not moving despite venous sticks for blood draw). I then call the patient by name, ask them to follow simple commands that represent high-yield tests differentiating the anterior from posterior symptoms (aphasia, inattention versus disconjugate gaze or ataxia), and check for extremity strength that was reported weak, as well as for gaze deviation or visual field loss, if any. As a result, I make a preliminarily determination of the following:

1. disabling deficit (yes, no, or symptoms resolved to a nondisabling level);

2. side of the brain lesion;

3. likely anterior versus posterior clinical lesion localization.

This determines my first step in the vascular ultrasound examination.

I start with the intracranial examination to locate the lesion or target vessel on the affected side [2], start monitoring the residual flow signals with the headframe [14], and then perform extracranial scanning [3]. Even though a lesion in the neck may be the source of the problem, the arterial obstruction that likely gives the patient the deficit is almost always located intracranially. Such clinically targeted, limited assessment can localize the lesion amenable to intervention within minutes. The protocols in Box 7.1 will explain in detail specific findings and differential diagnosis of a large variety of intracranial flow disturbances that could be found in the emergent situations.

Details of the Combined Extra-Intracranial Fast Track Insonation Protocol [3] are provided in Box 7.1. Specific depth ranges and insonation steps were first developed for nonimaging TCD but could also be used for motion-mode or image guided examinations [15].

Box 7.1 Fast track insonation protocol for TCD and carotid/ vertebral duplex

A. Clinical diagnosis of cerebral ischemia in the anterior circulation

Step 1: Transcranial Doppler

1. If time permits, begin insonation on the **nonaffected side** to establish the temporal window, normal MCA waveform (M1 depth 40–65 mm, M2 <30–40 mm) and velocity for comparison to the affected side.

2. If short on time, start on the **affected side**: first assess M1 MCA at 50 mm. If no signals detected, increase the depth to 60–65 mm (I usually set it at 64 mm – this depth range corresponds to the location of the most vessels comprising the circle of Willis: proximal MCA, TICA, A1 ACA, PCommA, and PCA. Therefore, the yield of finding a window of insonation is the highest here. If an antegrade flow signal is found, reduce the depth to trace the MCA stem distally until M2 segments are found, or identify the worst residual flow signal. Remember, "go with the flow" and explore all depth ranges

instead of stopping at easier detectable flow signals. It is counterintuitive but duplex imaging (and TCD) display better open vessels with more flow while the aim of an emergent examination is exactly the opposite: find arteries with the most reduced flow. In addition to surveying the affected artery, search for possible flow diversion to the ACA, PCA, or M2 MCA. Evaluate and compare waveform shapes and systolic flow acceleration.

3. Continue on the **affected side** (transorbital window). Check flow direction and pulsatility in the ophthalmic artery (OA) at depths of 40–50 mm, followed by ICA siphon at depths of 55–65 mm.

4. If time permits or in patients with pure motor or sensory deficits, evaluate BA (depth 80–100+ mm) and terminal VA (40–80 mm). Remember to use middle as well as lateral aspects of the foraminal window if the first probe placement yields only segmental detection of the vertebrobasilar system.

(Continued)

Explore all depth ranges where vessels are expected to be found and avoid crossing the midline in order not to sample the same VA twice.

Step 2: Carotid/ vertebral duplex

1. Start on the **affected side** in transverse B-mode planes followed by color or power-mode sweep from proximal to distal carotid segments. Identify CCA and its bifurcation on B-mode and flow-carrying lumens.

2. Document if the ICA (or CCA) has a lesion on B-mode and corresponding disturbances on flow images. In patients with concomitant chest pain, evaluate CCA as close to the origin as possible (look for possible intimal flaps in rare cases of aortic dissections).

3. Perform angle-corrected spectral velocity measurements in the mid-to-distal CCA, ICA, and ECA (the latter is necessary if a high-resistance flow is found in the ICA or vessel identification is uncertain during this brief assessment).

4. If time permits or in patients with pure motor or sensory deficits, examine the cervical portion of the vertebral arteries (longitudinal B-mode, color or power mode, spectral Doppler) on the **affected side**.

5. If time permits, perform transverse and longitudinal scanning of the arteries on the **nonaffected side** (particularly in patients with posterior circulation symptoms, examine the vertebral artery on the presumably nonaffected side because the often dominant vertebral artery can be the source of contralateral ischemic symptoms or bilateral posterior circulation strokes).

B. Clinical diagnosis of cerebral ischemia in the posterior circulation

Step 1: Transcranial Doppler

1. Start suboccipital insonation at 75 mm (VA junction) – this depth offers the highest yield of detection of the foraminal window as flow signals from both VAs and the proximal BA can be found there. Once the window is located, identify BA flow at 80–100+ mm.

2. If abnormal signals present at 75–100 mm, find the terminal VA (40–80 mm) on the nonaffected side for comparison and evaluate the terminal VA on the affected side at similar depths. Always remember that one vertebral artery may anatomically end in the posterior inferior cerebral artery (PICA) and may be noncontributory to the BA flow. Also remember that thrombi may propagate acutely and may be at this moment located in the vertebral artery segment after the PICA origin. Finally, if a dominate VA steno-occlusive lesion is suspected, check for possible retrograde flow in the distal BA from the anterior circulation or sluggish antegrade BA flow and cross-cerebellar collateralization.

3. Continue with transtemporal examination to identify PCA, focusing first on P1 and its origin (55–75 mm), identify the top of the basilar when possible (70–80 mm), and possible collateral flow through the posterior communicating artery (check both sides). Then proceed to evaluate for P2 PCA flow if PCA ischemia is suspected.

4. If time permits, evaluate both MCAs and ACAs (60–75 mm) for possible compensatory velocity increase as an indirect sign of the basilar artery obstruction.

Step 2: Vertebral/ carotid duplex ultrasound

1. Start on the affected side by locating the CCA using longitudinal B-mode plane and turn the transducer laterally and downward to visualize shadows from transverse processes of midcervical vertebrae.

2. Apply color or power modes and spectral Doppler to identify flow within intratransverse VA segments.

3. Follow the VA course to its origin and obtain Doppler spectra. Perform a similar examination on another side.

4. If time permits, perform bilateral duplex examination of the CCA, ICA, and ECA as described above.

References

1. Brott T, Adams HP Jr, Olinger CP, *et al.* Measurements of acute cerebral infarction: a clinical examination scale. *Stroke* 1989; **20**: 864–70.

2. Alexandrov AV, Demchuk A, Wein T, *et al.* The yield of transcranial Doppler in acute cerebral ischemia. *Stroke* 1999; **30**: 1605–9.

3. Chernyshev OY, Garami Z, Calleja S, *et al.* The yield and accuracy of urgent combined carotid-transcranial ultrasound testing in acute cerebral ischemia. *Stroke* 2005; **36**: 32–7.

4. Tsivgoulis G, Sharma VK, Lao AY, *et al.* Validation of transcranial Doppler with computed tomography angiography in acute cerebral ischemia. *Stroke* 2007; **38**: 1245–9.

5. Tsivgoulis G, Sharma VK, Hoover SL, *et al.* Applications and advantages of power motion-mode Doppler in acute posterior circulation cerebral ischemia. *Stroke* 2008; **39**: 1197–204.

6. Alexandrov AV. *Cerebrovascular Ultrasound in Stroke Prevention and Treatment*, 2nd edn. Oxford: Wiley-Blackwell, 2011.

7. Valdueza JM, Shreiber SJ, Roehl JE, *et al. Neurosonology and Neuroimaging of Stroke*. Stuttgart, Germany: Thieme, 2008.

8. Bartels E. *Color-Coded Duplex Ultrasonography of the Cerebral Arteries: Atlas and Manual*. Stuttgart, Germany: Schattauer, 1999.

9. Pellerito J, Polak J (eds). *Introduction to Vascular Ultrasonography*, 6th edn. Philedelphia: Saunders, 2012.

10. von Reutern GM, Budingen HJ. *Ultrasound Diagnosis of Cerebrovascular Disease*. Stuttgart: Georg Thieme Verlag, 1993.

11. AbuRahma AF, Pollack JA, Robinson PA, *et al*. The reliability of color duplex ultrasound in diagnosing total carotid artery occlusion. *Am J Surg* 1997; **174**: 185–7.

12. Demchuk AM, Christou I, Wein TH, *et al*. Specific transcranial Doppler flow findings related to the presence and site of arterial occlusion with transcranial Doppler. *Stroke* 2000; **31**: 140–6.

13. El-Mitwalli A, Saad M, Christou I, *et al*. Clinical and sonographic patterns of tandem ICA/MCA occlusion in TPA treated patients. *Stroke* 2002; **33**: 99–102.

14. Alexandrov AV, Demchuk AM, Felberg RA, *et al*. High rate of complete recanalization and dramatic clinical recovery during TPA infusion when continuously monitored by 2 MHz transcranial Doppler monitoring. *Stroke* 2000; **31**: 610–14.

15. Alexandrov AV, Sloan MA, Wong LKS, *et al*. Practice standards for transcranial Doppler (TCD) ultrasound. Part I. Test performance. *J Neuroimaging* 2007; **17**: 11–18.

8 Diagnostic Waveforms and Algorithms

"The Doppler waveform never lies. It is our own inability to understand its language that is the problem."
Merill P. Spencer, MD, pioneer in cerebrovascular ultrasound.

Deciphering the meaning of a few velocity data could be difficult if the rest of the ultrasound findings are not taken into account. Real-time blood flow traces and sounds immerse the physician into the wealth of pathophysiological information. This chapter will explain the waveform analysis and diagnostic algorithms I use to interpret both carotid duplex and transcranial Doppler findings. Velocity data come from the waveforms while the real depth of information within the waveforms and flow spectra remains to be explored.

For its normal function, the brain needs a continuous blood flow supply throughout the cardiac cycle and its delivery is governed by cerebral autoregulation. By comparing my sonographic findings to catheter angiograms carried out close together in time, I first learned what the real-time waveforms can start to tell us. I use the following specific steps to structure the analysis and interpretation of waveforms [1]:

Step 1. Identify the beginning and the end of a single cardiac cycle (Figure 8.1).

Step 2. Determine the following aspects:

i. sharpness of the systolic flow acceleration;

ii. the end-diastolic flow consistent with the expected resistance in the arterial system supplied by the sampled vessel;

iii. waveform shape transmission from the proximal to the distal part of the vessel;

iv. symmetry with the contralateral homologous segment; and

v. the presence of any cardiac, systemic, or focal circulatory condition(s) that could explain the waveform.

Step 3. Synthesize the information and explain the waveform appearance as attributable to:

i. technical error or an artifact;

ii. systemic hemodynamic conditions;

iii. the presence of a focal lesion;

iv. increased, normal, or decreased intracranial resistance.

Waveforms discussed below represent typical findings to illustrate this algorithm.

Waveforms in vessels with normal patency

Various waveforms can be obtained from vessels with normal patency. They represent a wide spectrum of what constitutes normal findings or correspond to a normal local patency on angiography in the precerebral vessels (Figure 8.2). Intracranial waveforms can be even more diverse.

Sharp (or vertical) systolic flow acceleration implies that the blood pool reached the insonated vessel with no delays. It will not be affected by an obstruction distal to the site of insonation and it implies that the proximal vessels are likely patent. Systolic flow acceleration can still be sharp (or look normal) in some patients with severe proximal steno-occlusive lesions, and this finding in a vessel distal to such a significant obstruction implies brisk collaterals.

A sharp systolic acceleration can still be present with **congestive heart failure** (CHF). In this case, the peak systolic complex appears smaller, and this could make one suspect a blunted signal (i.e. a delayed systolic flow acceleration, which will be discussed below) (Figure 8.3). Looking at other vessel waveforms, particularly on the contralateral side, can help

Neurovascular Examination: The Rapid Evaluation of Stroke Patients Using Ultrasound Waveform Interpretation, First Edition.
Andrei V. Alexandrov.
© 2013 Andrei V. Alexandrov. Published 2013 by Blackwell Publishing Ltd.

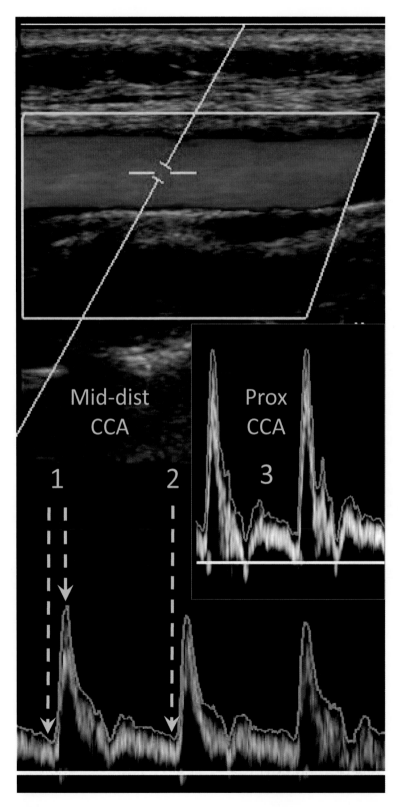

Mid-dist CCA

Prox CCA

1   2

3

Figure 8.1 CCA waveform with phases of cardiac cycle. 1, early systolic upstroke; 2, end-diastoli; 3, diastolic phase after the closure of the aortic valve (flow deceleration to zero with short reversal that could be seen in the CCA).

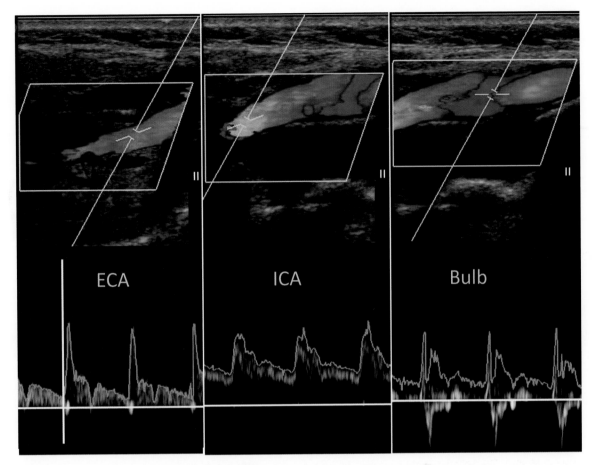

Figure 8.2 Typical waveforms in the bulb, ICA, and ECA.

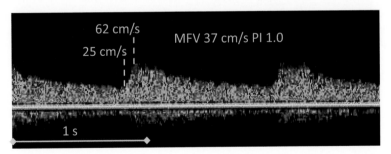

Figure 8.3 Waveform in a patient with CHF and normal M1 MCA patency. Note the low-velocity systolic flow acceleration making the systolic complex less prominent.

with this differential. In cases when a heart condition leads to changes in hemodynamics of the cerebral vessels, similar waveforms are seen bilaterally and in both the anterior and posterior circulations. Also, knowing the cardiac output, ejection fraction, and systolic/ diastolic blood pressures could be helpful to determine what changes are largely driven by the heart and what is more reflective of local hemodynamic conditions.

Flow velocity deceleration and end-diastolic velocities are largely determined by a combination of the cardiac function, local vessel compliance, and distal resistance. Knowing if a patient has chronic or systolic hypertension, diffuse atheromatous disease, or if a vessel supplies a high-resistance bed (i.e. ECA) provides clues to the shape of the waveform. Figures 8.1 and 8.2 show the waveform follower, or envelope, that outlines the maximum frequencies in the spectral Doppler. If gain settings are correct, the envelope outlines the waveform shape after the peak systolic rise, flow deceleration, and the proportion of the end-diastolic flow component.

Further consideration should be given to vessel diameter changes, such as at the level of the **carotid bulb** (Figure 8.2). Natural vessel dilations lead to flow separation or reversal and can result in a variety of waveforms ranging from slow antegrade flow to a more complex bidirectional waveforms or having areas with flow reversal that could appear to be high resistance. In case of the carotid bulb waveform, this flow reversal occurs at low blood flow velocities which exposes vessel walls to a low shear stress, factors that predispose to atherogenesis at this site and its geometry is implicated as a risk factor [2, 3]. Comparison of these waveforms to B-mode image and adjustment of color flow velocity scale can help identify these waveforms as reflecting normal vessel patency. These waveforms could be confusing if these are the only ones obtainable at the ICA origin in patients with so-called high bifurcations (where access to the ICA is limited by the jaw). Looking at the CCA waveforms and extending investigation of the distal ICA on the neck could help avoid this confusion. Several further steps can be taken here, including duplex scanning with a posterior approach and the patient's head turned up and away from the interrogated side, as well as insonation with a nonimaging 2-MHz Doppler from beneath the jaw at a depth of 30–60 mm or with tran-

soral application of duplex imaging using a different transducer [4–6].

Interpretation of diverse hemodynamically driven findings requires consideration of whether the detected changes are due to systemic, focal precerebral, or intracranial factors. In a case where the blood flow is affected by cardiac output and viscosity, expect the waveform changes to be equally represented in both affected and nonaffected vessels, bilaterally and in both the anterior and posterior circulation vessels. Symmetry is applicable not only to the velocity data but also to the shape of the waveforms. In fact, the velocities could be different but the waveforms may look alike – this makes me suspect the angle of vessel intercept to be primarily responsible for the velocity asymmetry. In addition to thinking about the usual suspects (errors, artifacts, anatomy), documentation of the circulatory conditions that can affect the waveforms and velocities is an important part of neurovascular ultrasound examination.

I often look at just waveforms themselves before I take into account the velocity changes. Take for example **atrial fibrillation** (AFib) (Figure 8.4): the peak systolic complexes can be quite variable in amplitude. Some peak systolic complexes can be disproportionately high. However, the diastolic flow remains relatively low but steady. Patients with AFib can have overall normal or low velocities and high pulsatility index (PI) just because our calculation methods that average over several seconds do not take into account variability of the cardiac output with more or less synchronous atrial fillings. Note that the key feature of the waveform from the MCA with normal patency in a patient with AFib is the continuous diastolic flow despite variability of the systolic supply. The brain adjusts by vasodilation to make sure that even with the lowest cardiac output, it still receives a steady blood supply. This is how the brain ensures constant delivery of cerebral blood flow despite malfunction of the pump.

Similarly with **aortic valve insufficiency** (Figure 8.4b), a transient reversal of flow at the time of the aortic valve closure is seen in the terminal ICA/MCA origin. This reversal disappears in the proximal MCA, although dicrotic flow deceleration remains quite prominent.

Another systemic condition that is useful to keep in mind because it affects the waveform is **anemia** (Figure 8.5). Changes to hematocrit, viscosity, and

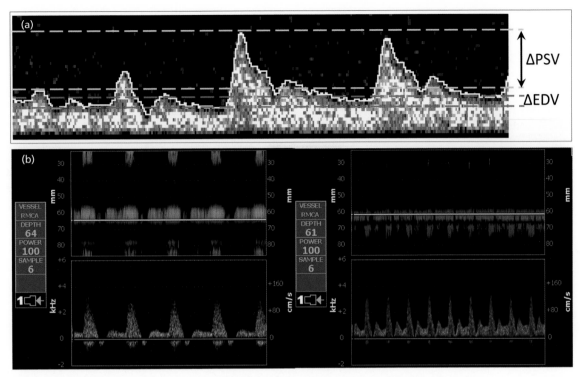

Figure 8.4 Waveforms with atrial fibrillation (**a**) and aortic valve insufficiency (**b**). Both were obtained in patients with normal MCA patency.

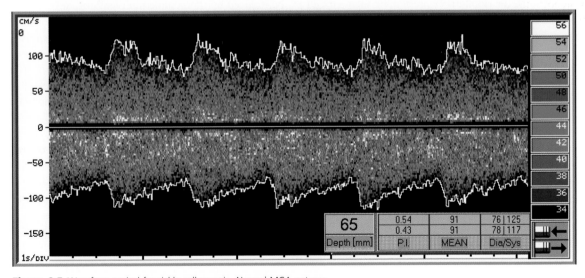

Figure 8.5 Waveform typical for sickle cell anemia. Normal MCA patency.

oxygen-carrying capacity are at play, leading to a specific pattern: abundance of the diastolic flow because brain needs more blood flow volume delivered in a unit of time to compensate for fewer oxygen-carrying cells. This is indirectly evident from a disproportionately high diastolic flow velocity and resulting low PIs.

The caveat here is that a similar waveform can be present with an increased flow volume in patients with normal oxygen -carrying capacity. A drop in resistance to flow will allow higher diastolic velocities that may have no abnormal correlate (i.e. vasodilation with hypoventilation) or may be present with structural lesions such as an arteriovenous malformation (AVM, feeding vessel) or AV fistulae. All of these can lead to an artificial rise in EDV. All can have bruits within the waveform, and these are not helpful to differentiate these conditions from the effects of anemia.

A quick look at an arterial segment proximal to the site of insonation and at the homologous contralateral vessel will provide the answers. With anemia, velocities are high everywhere and PIs are low due to compensatory vasodilation that lowers the resistance, attracts more flow per unit of time, and delivers the amount of oxygen tissues usually need. With a shunt such as AVM or fistulae, the findings are focal and found on the side of the feeding vessel. With an arterial stenosis, the proximal or prestenotic segment will have normal or low velocities with normal or high PIs. In addition, try to sample the poststenotic segment.

A specific condition called **hyperemia** will produce a unique pattern of high-velocity–low-resistance waveforms (Figure 8.6) in one artery or one system depending on the cause, while the remainder of the vessels may have normal velocities and PIs. The latter can be seen with the hyperdynamic states following subarachnoid hemorrhage (SAH) [7], hyperperfusion syndrome post carotid revascularization [8], systemic tPA therapy, or intra-arterial reperfusion [9]. Caution should be exercised when applying traditional velocity/ ratio criteria as TCD predictions of blood flow changes may not correlate with other cerebral blood flow measuring techniques in patients with SAH [7]. Other areas have more robust diagnostic criteria for hyperemia [8, 9].

Other conditions that can significantly affect the waveforms are **infections** (Figure 8.6). Patients with infections often have hyperdynamic states that cause the brain to respond with vasoconstriction. As a result, the waveform becomes more pulsatile. Despite PI values suggestive of high resistance and possibly increased intracranial pressure (i.e. PI values $\geq$ 1.2), the **systemic vascular resistance** (SVR) is actually low and PIs should not be over-interpreted in the presence of a wide-spread infection.

It is important to understand that in response to a drop in blood pressure (BP), cardiac output, or a vessel occlusion with a balloon, normal autoregulation in the brain will induce vasodilation and decrease the resistance to flow (Figure 8.7). The result will be maintenance of the cerebral blood flow while the waveform will have lower velocities and lower PIs, while systolic acceleration will depend on the presence or absence of a focal obstruction to flow causing distal pressure drop. SVR governs the rest of the body and it reacts in the opposite way: low BP causes SVR to raise through peripheral vasoconstriction. In a case of infection, these adjustments become more complex and multifactorial. A decrease in SVR results in reduced systemic flow. This combined with tachycardia decreases diastolic heart filling, further reducing the diastolic pressure. The resulting brain waveforms could be affected by these systemic factors as well as preservation or decompensation of autoregulatory mechanisms.

Some of the changes in the arterial waveforms can be induced by therapeutic interventions. Several cardiology devices could be applied in patients with concomitant cerebrovascular disease based on clinical indications such as heart failure, myocardial infarction, etc. [10]. Figure 8.8a shows a waveform in a patient with patent MCA who received a mistimed **intra-aortic balloon pump** (IABP) to augment diastolic flow to the heart. Note the brief flow gaps in the MCA waveform at mistimed deflations. Figure 8.8b shows a properly ECG-triggered **external counter-pulsation** (ECP) device that squeezes the lower extremities and causes flow diversion in diastoli to both the heart (not shown) and brain [11]. Note the appearance of the peak augmented diastolic component, termed PDAV, which is higher than peak systoli in a healthy volunteer. Figure 8.8c shows the MCA flow profile in a patient with a **left ventricular assist device** (LVAD).

Waveforms often give me a clue as to what is likely happening systemically, or locally, or both. Subsequent velocity, ratio, and other data analyses provide

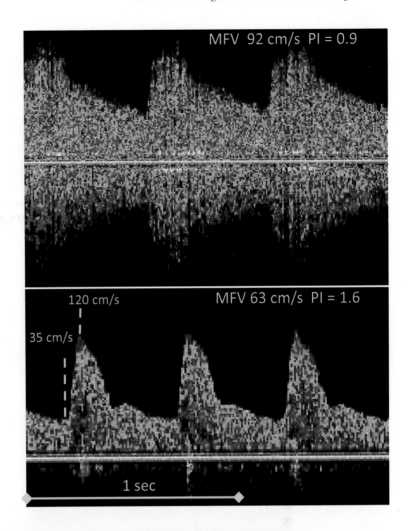

MFV 92 cm/s PI = 0.9

120 cm/s

35 cm/s

MFV 63 cm/s PI = 1.6

1 sec

Figure 8.6 Waveforms from patent MCAs in patients with hyperemia and hyperdynamic states (i.e. infection).

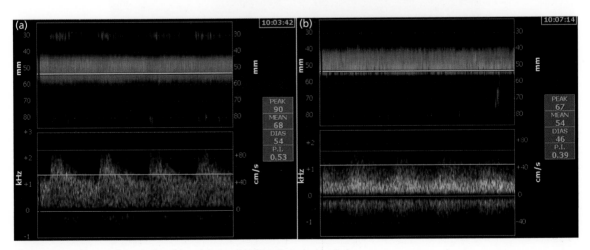

Figure 8.7 MCA waveforms before (**a**) and during (**b**) ICA balloon test occlusion.

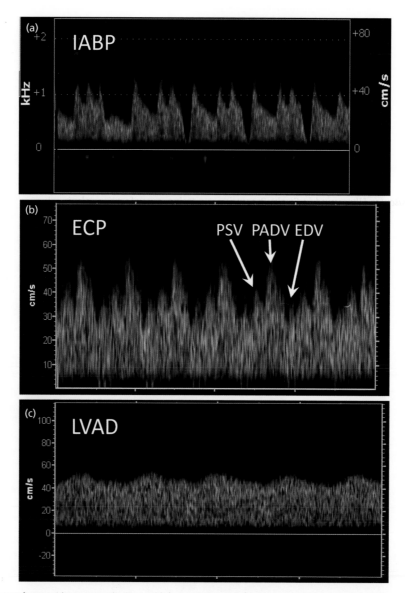

Figure 8.8 MCA waveforms with counterpulsation and left ventricular assist devices: (**a**) IABP, intra-aortic balloon pump; (**b**) ECP, external counter pulsation; PADV, peak augmented diastolic velocity; (**c**) LVAD, left ventricular assist device. All waveforms were obtained from MCAs with normal patency.

support for diagnostic considerations and more objective interpretation of test results.

When looking at the waveform, I ask myself how will the insonated vessel look on a catheter angiogram if dye is injected directly into it. Thus, there could be three answers:

1. normal patency,
2. stenosis, or
3. occlusion.

Findings that are associated with patent vessels are as discussed above, and additional discussion can be found in *Cerebrovascular Ultrasound in Stroke Prevention and Treatment* – chapter on Practical Models of Cerebral Hemodynamics and Waveform Recognition [12]. Spectral waveforms that correlate with normal patency at the site of insonation in the presence of collaterals or flow reversal will be discussed as part of diagnostic algorithms and differential diagnoses. Waveforms that reflect abnormal patency of the vasculature will be analyzed in the rest of this chapter.

Waveforms indicating abnormalities in the vasculature

When vessel patency is likely compromised, the question I ask about any given waveform or other findings is: if there is a lesion, where is it on the **Spencer's curve** [13] (Figure 8.9), that is on the upslope or on the "other" side [14]? In other words, what is happening with the hemodynamics of the vessel? This will have implications for the next set of more specific questions, which address the clinical significance of ultrasound findings: is it less than 50% diameter reduction, or is it greater than 50%? If greater than 50%, is it greater than 70%? And furthermore, is it hemodynamically significant, that is comparable to a stenosis reducing the diameter by ≥80% ? Or is this a near-occlusive lesion? Or do I also see changes consistent with other processes such as hypo- or hyperperfusion, embolization, steal, etc.

Waveforms may remain low resistance, or show signs of artificially low resistance despite the degree of obstruction – reasons for this include the fact that diastolic flow may persevere across the lesion or around it through collaterals. If the patient remains asymptomatic, cerebral blood flow is still enough to avoid neuronal malfunction despite the presence of abnormal waveforms. Yet their presence tells me that this balance is fragile and may not be sustained for long. Once the patient becomes symptomatic, it signifies that the blood flow is being depleted, and these waveforms point to the likely mechanism and the source – is there hypoperfusion, reocclusion, or steal, and where are they coming from? This is why the velocity cannot be equated to flow volume, and this is also why the pulsatility index may not detect or explain the entire spectrum of arterial lesions. While I acknowledge these caveats, I also believe that qualitative waveform analysis along with the velocity, overall pulsatility, ratios, and flow diversion assessments can provide a fairly accurate estimate of the obstruction presence and severity in a given vessel. On the other hand, careful analysis may also determine whether there are other mechanisms of brain damage at play beyond the obstruction.

Blood is a non-Newtonian fluid, and waveforms are a reflection of its adaptation to the degree of stenosis, thus providing additional information from our velocity/ ratio measurements. In the future, more quantitative information should be derived from waveform and spectral analyses as our hemodynamic models are integrated with advances in imaging, mathematics, and computational capabilities. The waveforms may also contain information about laminar versus disturbed/ turbulent nature of blood flow that are atheroprotective and atherogenic, respectively. This information could be useful in future studies of endothelial function and to individualize the risk of atheroma formation and progression.

Waveforms on the upslope of the Spencer's curve can be quite variable but most of them carry similar themes (Figure 8.9). Velocities are mostly within the normal range for a given vessel in patients who are older than young adults (e.g. MCA MFV 30–80 cm/s), or are slightly to significantly elevated (e.g. adult MCA MFV values for any stenosis, ≥80 cm/s; for ≥50% stenosis, ≥100 cm/s). Velocities could be relatively low if the hematocrit is high [15], cardiac output is low, or the patient is elderly [16]. Ratios with the feeding vessels or homologous segments remain low or predictably high within ranges of the velocity increase corresponding to moderate (e.g. ICA/CCA PSV ratio 2.0 to <4.0 for ICA) and severe (≥4.0 for ≥70% ICA stenosis) disease processes [17, 18]. Changes in the diastolic flow are mostly determined by the degree of

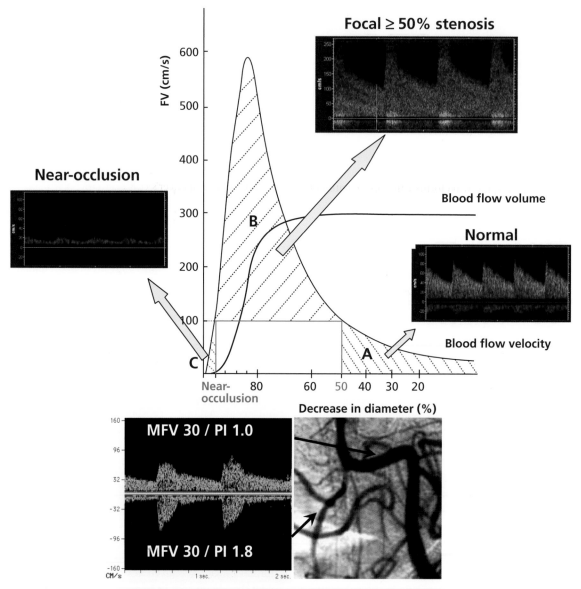

Figure 8.9 Waveforms on the upslope and the other side of the Spencer's curve. From right to left, the upslope of the Spencer's curve has normal velocity/ low-resistance waveform (A) and a stenotic waveform with increased PSV, bruit, and EDV found with the increasing degree of the stenosis (B). On the left, there is an example of the waveform from the "other" side of the Spencer's curve, i.e. the downslope where despite the increasing critical degree of the stenosis, the velocity decreases being falsely within the normal range (C), and waveform morphology can change. The insert below the graph shows two terminal vertebral artery waveforms obtained at the same time using a single Doppler gate at their junction: the antegrade flow towards the brain (away from the probe, inverted image – waveform above the baseline) has a low-resistance, normal-velocity waveform on the upslope of the Spencer's curve. It originates from the right VA that has a normal diameter on the catheter angiogram and supplies the basilar artery. The retrograde flow towards the probe (below the baseline) is from the reversed left terminal VA that on the angiogram has a small caliper and is affected by a long narrowing caused by either hypoplasia or vasospasm. Nonetheless, the shape of the waveform shows a high-resistance pattern and indicates overall hemodynamic significance of the lesion (i.e. placing this waveform on the "other side" of the Spencer's curve).

the stenosis at the severe end of its spectrum, cardiac function, and, in case of intracranial vessels, risk factors such as chronic hypertension [19], which produces greater vessel stiffness and higher PI values but not necessarily lesions that are detectable and measurable with current ultrasound methods.

Waveforms on the other side of the Spencer's curve are less predictable and more striking. In the precerebral vessels, several terms describe the waveforms [1]: pulse could be tardus parvus, end-diastolic flow may be greatly diminished or absent, and drum-like/ short systolic spike waveforms can appear with complete distal occlusion or near occlusion (Figure 8.10). If somewhat elevated velocity waveforms across the

lesion are found, these may yield unexpectedly high velocity ratios with the feeding vessel.

In the intracranial vasculature, changes in the waveforms along the Spencer's curve are described by the Thrombolysis in Brain Ischemia (TIBI) residual flow grading scale (the waveforms and corresponding angiograms can be found in Chapter 6) [20, 21]. **TIBI flow grades** indicating a complete or partial occlusion (TIBI 0–3) are attributable to the other side of the Spencer's curve, whereas the TIBI grades 4 and 5 correspond to the stenotic and normal parts on the upslope of the Spencer's curve.

Analogous to the Thrombolysis in Myocardial Infarction (TIMI) flow grades, TIBI waveforms predict

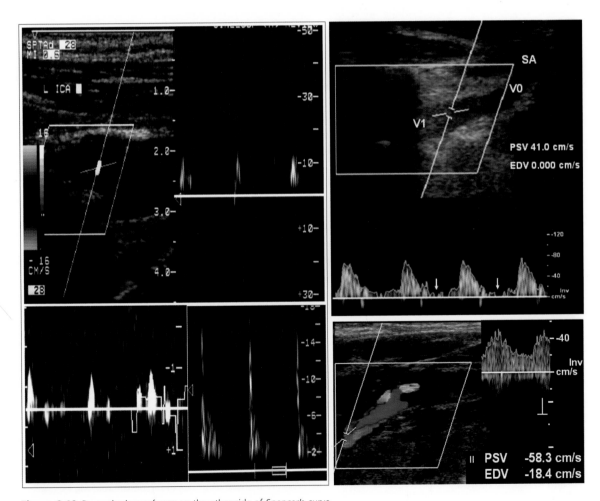

Figure 8.10 Precerebral waveforms on the other side of Spencer's curve.

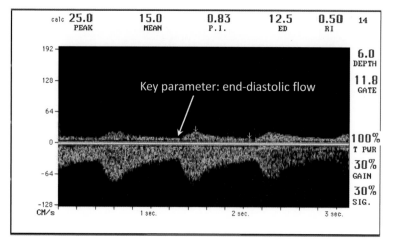

| calc 25.0 PEAK | 15.0 MEAN | 0.83 P.I. | 12.5 ED | 0.50 RI | 14 |

Key parameter: end-diastolic flow

6.0 DEPTH
11.8 GATE
100% T PWR
30% GAIN
30% SIG.

Figure 8.11 Typical waveforms at the terminal ICA bifurcation with MCA occlusion. Note blunted signal with positive EDV and flow diversion to ACA (i.e. MFV ACA > MCA).

intracranial vessel patency on catheter angiography. Absent and minimal waveforms (TIBI 0–1) predict a complete TIMI 0–I occlusion, blunted and dampened waveforms (TIBI 2–3) correlate with persisting or partial occlusions with TIMI IIa–b flow, and stenotic and normal waveforms (TIBI 4–5) indicate complete focal recanalization with TIMI III tissue reperfusion with or without a residual stenosis. The end-diastolic flow velocity is the key component (Figure 8.11) that allows prediction of local recanalization [22] in good-to-excellent agreement with catheter angiography [23]. Persistent occlusion and the no-reflow phenomenon are associated with absent or low end-diastolic flow velocities, such as seen with TIBI 0–1 and 2–3 waveforms. However, a modest EDV recovery during reperfusion therapies is generally predictive of at least TIMI II flow or better and a greater chance of earlier and faster neurological recovery.

Steps to determine TIBI flow grades: A specific algorithm (designed while at the University of Texas with my colleagues Andrew Demchuk and Scott Burgin) should be applied when learning how to identify those waveforms (copyright: Health Outcomes Institute, 2000; reproduced with permission):

1. Comparison (or nonaffected*) side: evaluate waveform shape and determine systolic acceleration, velocity, and pulsatility of flow.

2. Affected side: analyze differences in the waveform shape by determining end-diastolic velocity (EDV):

if none → minimal or absent signals;

if present → other signals below.

3. If EDV is present: loss or flattening of the peak systolic complex and PI <1.2 indicates a blunted signal.
4. If the systolic acceleration is normal (sharp upstroke) and mean velocity is decreased by 30% or more relative to the comparison side, this indicates a dampened signal.
5. If MFV is ≥80 cm/s and/or ≥30% higher than the comparison side, then the stenotic signal is present (also note other signs of the stenosis like the presence of turbulence; bruits can be present with both stenosis and normal hyperemic signals).
6. If the differences between the sides are within 30% and the systolic acceleration upstrokes are similar, a normal signal is present.

Figures 8.12, 8.13, 8.14, 8.15, 8.16 and 8.17 show typical examples of these waveforms in relationship to the nonaffected vessel waveforms that should be used for comparison.

---

* For the basilar artery waveforms, use nonaffected vertebral artery if available, or one of the nonaffected MCAs.

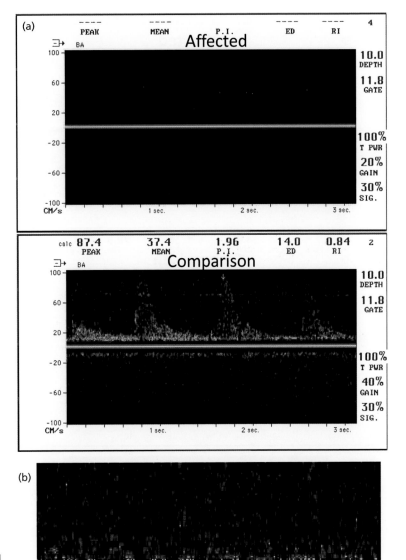

Figure 8.12 (a) Absent flow signal. No flow signals were obtained. Absent signal is diagnosed only if background noise and no regular pulsations are seen throughout the recording time (b).

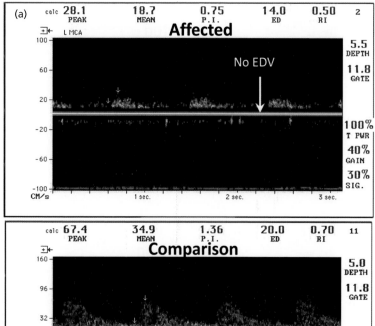

(a)

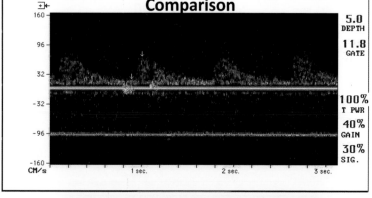

(b)

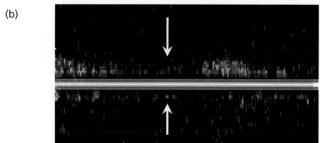

Figure 8.13 (**a**) Minimal flow signal. No end-diastolic flow is found. Only peak systolic spikes (of variable velocities) are present. Background noise can be mistaken for end-diastolic signals. (**b**) Noise signals present in diastoli above and below baseline. As a rule we do not undergain spectral window and do not use low-frequency filters. Therefore some noise is expected to be present through diastoli and it is infrequently a "judgment" or subjective call. Usually when true diastolic signals are present, they are present more consistently on one side of the baseline while the other side has more intermittent noise signals.

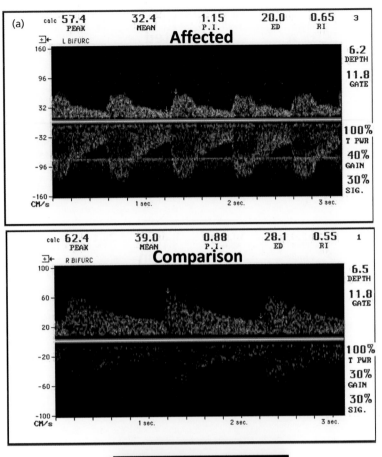

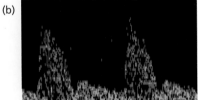

Figure 8.14 (**a**) Blunted flow signal. Flattening or loss of peak systoli results in delayed flow acceleration and less pulsatile waveform shape with positive EDV and low PI of 0.83. Normal signal differs from blunted by initial sharp systolic upstroke even if later flow deceleration may be slow. Both waveforms in (**b**) are normal.

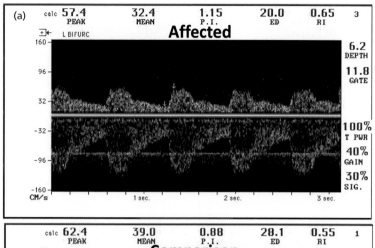

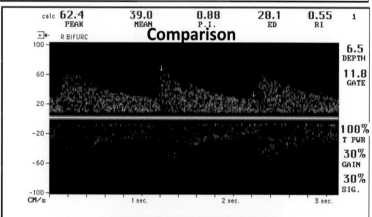

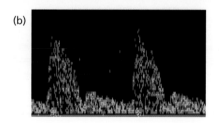

Figure 8.15 (a) Dampened flow signal. Sharp systolic upstroke and pulsatile waveform (*shape* and PI 1.15 vs. 0.88 of comparison side). Also note flow diversion to ACA (MFV ACA below baseline > MCA). Flow velocities may be within 30% difference between the sides. Note pulsatile shape of the waveform in (**b**); the difference in pulsatility may be the only indicator of a persisting distal or branch occlusion.

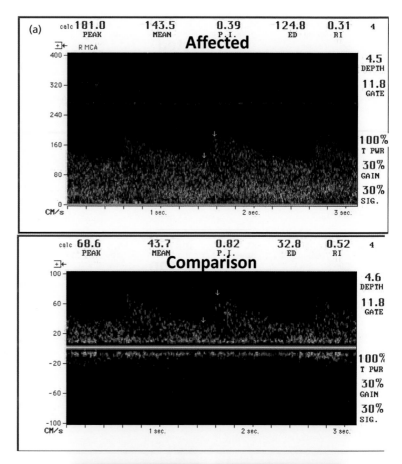

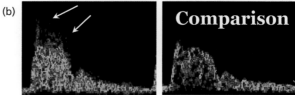

Figure 8.16 (**a**) Stenotic flow signal. Unilateral mean velocity increase MCA ≥ 80 cm/s and/or ≥ 30% difference with comparison side. Low EDV may decrease MFV values. Look for other signs of stenosis such as turbulence (arrows) in (**b**).

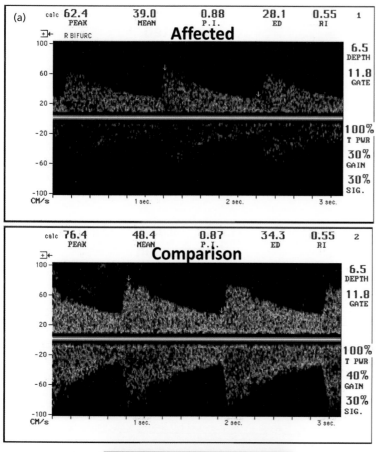

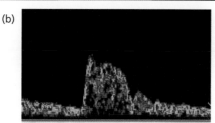

Figure 8.17 (**a**) Normal flow signal. Flow waveforms are similar in shape including systolic upstroke and EDV. Flow velocities are within 30% difference between sides. Note that EDV may be low in hypertensive patients and waveforms can appear as high resistance bilaterally (**b**).

There are waveforms however that, at first glance, are difficult to classify into any specific TIBI grade (Figure 8.18). This figure depicts the presence of turbulence with an embolus that causes a high-grade stenosis in the distal M1 segment of the MCA. This is a lesion on the other side of the Spencer's curve as evident from a disturbed waveform, lower than expected elevation of the systolic velocity, and low end-diastolic flow. Note that this patient was still

having disabling symptoms at the time when this waveform was detected. This is a TIBI grade IV stenotic signal (Figure 8.18a). The waveform below (Figure 8.18b) was obtained in the same patient when the distal M1 MCA embolus started to recanalize during treatment with intravenous tPA and it moved to the proximal M2 MCA. As a result, a dampened TIBI III waveform appeared as compared to the nonaffected side (data not shown). However, it still has the

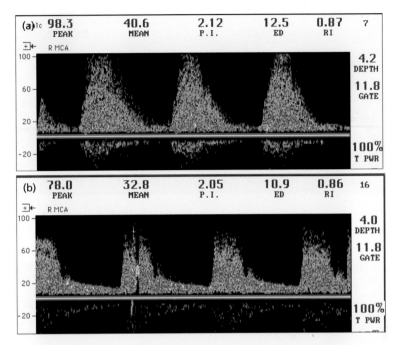

Figure 8.18 Atypical TIBI waveforms I.
(**a**) TIBI 4 stenotic signal; (**b**) TIBI 3
dampened or suppressed signal with signs
of turbulence (more explanations are
provided in the text).

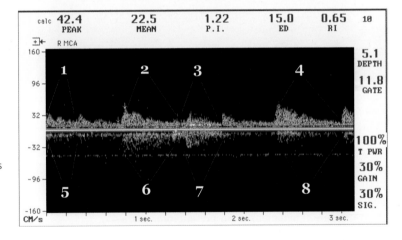

Figure 8.19 Atypical TIBI waveforms II.
1,TIBI 3 dampened signal; 2, TIBI 3
dampened; 3, TIBI 2 blunted (with
high-intensity signals suggesting thrombus
propagation); 4, TIBI 3 dampened; 5, TIBI
2 blunted; 6, TIBI 2 blunted (with
turbulence); 7, TIBI 3 dampened; 8, TIBI 1
minimal signal.

presence of turbulence and now shows a high-intensity transient embolic signal. These were indirect signs that residual embolic material could still be present in the M1 MCA or an additional and more proximal embolus could exist. Compared to baseline, both indicate recanalization and some degree of distal reperfusion. However, both should be interpreted with caution as there may still be a persisting hemodynamically significant partial obstruction to flow and even though the patient started to improve neurologically, he still

has not achieved complete reperfusion. This may account for some discrepancies between Doppler spectral assessment of flow and concurrent catheter angiographic assessments [23].

Figures 8.19, 8.20, and 8.21 further illustrate polymorphic waveform changes with thrombi propagation (Figure 8.19) and changes in blood pressure and proximal vessel patency with aortic dissection extending into both CCAs (Figures 8.20 and 8.21). The latter patient presented with the left-sided weakness and the

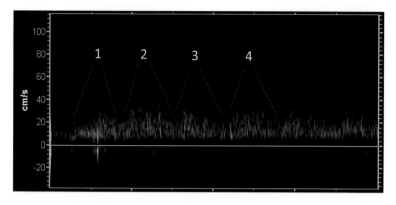

Figure 8.20 Atypical TIBI waveforms III. 1, TIBI 2 blunted signal with velocity improvement indicating either the beginning/ continuation of recanalization (including proximal recanalization) or improvement in the residual MCA flow with increasing blood pressure; 2, TIBI 3 dampened signal due to appearance of more vertical systolic upstroke; 3, TIBI 3 dampened; and 4, TIBI 2 blunted signals.

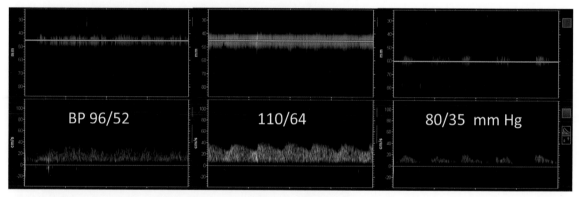

Figure 8.21 TIBI waveforms in the MCA with aortic arch dissection and acute stroke. Residual flow changes as follows (from let to right) TIBI 2-3-2-1. The presence of microemboli and a similar delay in systolic flow acceleration on the nonaffected side (images not shown) point to a proximal source obstruction such as the ascending aortic arch dissection.

waveforms were obtained in the right MCA during blood pressure fluctuations upon presentation at the Emergency Department.

These waveforms reflect flow dynamics to and around an acute thromboembolic occlusions. Because the majority of patients still arrive beyond the current window for reperfusion therapies or continue to have persisting occlusions despite treatment, ultrasound insights into how arterial blood flow is redistributed and how it responds to certain stimuli could form the basis for the development of novel flow augmentation therapies. The next chapter will address algorithms for differential diagnosis of ultrasound findings across a wide range of conditions.

References

1. Alexandrov AV. Extra- and intracranial waveform analysis algorithm, descriptions, classifications and differential diagnosis. *J Vasc Ultrasound* 2012; **36**: 103–12.
2. Nguyen KT, Clark CD, Chancellor TJ, *et al*. Carotid geometry effects on blood flow and on risk for vascular disease. *J Biomech* 2008; **41**: 11–19.
3. Sitzer M, Puac D, Buehler A, *et al*. Internal carotid artery angle of origin: a novel risk factor for early carotid atherosclerosis. *Stroke* 2003; **34**: 950–5.
4. Yasaka M, Kimura K, Otsubo R, *et al*. Transoral carotid ultrasonography. *Stroke* 1998; **29**: 1383–8.
5. Yakushiji Y, Takase Y, Kosugi M, *et al*. Transoral carotid ultrasonography is useful for detection and follow-up

of extracranial internal carotid artery dissecting aneurysm. *Cerebrovasc Dis* 2007; **24**: 144–6.

6. Suzuki R, Koga M, Toyoda K, *et al*. Identification of internal carotid artery dissection by transoral carotid ultrasonography. *Cerebrovasc Dis* 2012; **33**: 369–77.

7. Rothoerl RD, Woertgen C, Brawanski A. Hyperemia following aneurysmal subarachnoid hemorrhage: incidence, diagnosis, clinical features, and outcome. *Intensive Care Med* 2004; **30**: 1298–302.

8. Spencer MP. Transcranial Doppler monitoring and causes of stroke from carotid endarterectomy. *Stroke* 1997; **28**: 685–91.

9. Rubiera M, Cava L, Tsivgoulis G, *et al*. Diagnostic criteria and yield of real time transcranial Doppler (TCD) monitoring of intra-arterial (IA) reperfusion procedures. *Stroke* 2010; **41**: 695–9.

10. Brass LM. Reversed intracranial blood flow in patients with an intra-aortic balloon pump. *Stroke* 1990; **21**: 484–7.

11. Alexandrov AW, Ribo M, Wong KS, *et al*. Perfusion augmentation in acute stroke using mechanical counter-pulsation-Phase IIa. Effect of external counterpulsation on middle cerebral artery mean flow velocity in five healthy subjects. *Stroke* 2008; **39**: 2760–4.

12. Alexandrov AV. *Cerebrovascular Ultrasound in Stroke Prevention and Treatment*, 2nd edn. Oxford: Wiley-Blackwell, 2011.

13. Spencer MP, Reid JM. Quantitation of carotid stenosis with continuous wave Doppler ultrasound. *Stroke* 1979; **10**: 326–30.

14. Alexandrov AV. The Spencer's curve: clinical implications of a classic hemodynamic model. *J Neuroimaging* 2007; **17**: 6–10.

15. Brass LM, Pavlakis SG, DeVivo D, *et al*. Transcranial Doppler measurements of the middle cerebral artery. Effect of hematocrit. *Stroke* 1988; **19**: 1466–9.

16. Arnolds BJ, von Reutern GM. Transcranial Doppler sonography. Examination technique and normal reference values. *Ultrasound Med Biol* 1986; **12**: 115–23.

17. Grant EG, Benson, CB, Moneta, GL, *et al*. Carotid artery stenosis: gray-scale and Doppler US diagnosis – Society of Radiologists in Ultrasound Consensus Conference. *Radiology* 2003; **229**: 340–6.

18. von Reutern GM, Goertler MW, Bornstein NM, *et al*; Neurosonology Research Group of the World Federation of Neurology. Grading carotid stenosis using ultrasonic methods. *Stroke* 2012; **43**: 916–21.

19. Kidwell CS, el-Saden S, Livshits Z, *et al*. Transcranial Doppler pulsatility indices as a measure of diffuse small-vessel disease. *J Neuroimaging* 2001; **11**: 229–35.

20. Demchuk AM, Burgin WS, Christou I, *et al*. Thrombolysis in Brain Ischemia (TIBI) transcranial Doppler flow grades predict clinical severity, early recovery, and mortality in patients treated with tissue plasminogen activator. *Stroke* 2001; **32**: 89–93.

21. Alexandrov AV. Ultrasound-enhanced thrombolysis for stroke: clinical significance. *Eur J Ultrasound* 2002; **16**: 131–40.

22. Burgin WS, Malkoff M, Felberg RA, *et al*. Transcranial Doppler ultrasound criteria for recanalization after thrombolysis for middle cerebral artery stroke. *Stroke* 2000; **31**: 1128–32.

23. Tsivgoulis G, Ribo M, Rubiera M, *et al*. Real-time validation of transcranial Doppler criteria in assessing recanalization during intra-arterial procedures for acute ischemic stroke: an international, multicenter study. *Stroke* 2013; **44**: 394–400.

9   Differential Diagnosis

"Clinical correlation is advised."

Ubiqitous statement in test reports

Introduction

Technological progress increasingly provides more portable tools to image organs and evaluate systems at the bedside, in a fast and convenient manner. Signal optimization, data display, and incorporation of diagnostic criteria and automated differential algorithms will aid test interpretation. One of the major problems with transcranial Doppler interpretation is the vast differential diagnosis, while commonly used duplex criteria for grading carotid stenosis on the neck are often too simplistic [1]. For instance, consensus was obtained only for grading a short and unilateral stenosis [2], and even these criteria are now being questioned and multiparametric grading systems are advocated [3]. The challenge is how to interpret cerebrovascular ultrasound studies when many patients have findings outside the box: tandem lesions, bilateral disease, coexistence of systemic and focal abnormalities, hyperacute and often sudden hemodynamic changes, and the list goes on. This chapter will describe how I analyze an image or waveform obtained in a certain vessel, what specific findings I'm looking for next and where I look for these, and what conditions I suspect could produce these findings. Current diagnostic criteria and differential diagnosis will be discussed in the following sequence:

1. carotid artery stenosis
2. carotid artery occlusion
3. vertebral artery hypoplasia, stenosis, dissection, and occlusion
4. systemic and cardiac abnormalities that could affect differential diagnosis
5. downstream effects of carotid lesions
6. intracranial stenoses versus collaterals
7. intracranial occlusion localization
8. vasospasm
9. hyperemia
10. steal.

Carotid artery stenosis

Grading carotid stenosis with ultrasound relies on integration of several findings and should be multiparametric [3]. As scanning progresses or as you review consecutive images, pay attention to the B-mode for detection of any structural abnormality (intima–media thickening, formation of a fatty streak, plaque, or presence of a thrombus). If I see a lesion, I quickly eyeball it first to decide if it is causing less or greater than 50% diameter reduction. It is useful to see both longitudinal and transverse projections, as longitudinal near-wall views can overestimate mild plaque protrusion into the lumen while hypoechoic concentric and large plaques may look smaller than they really are on longitudinal views in B-mode only. I then proceed with a comparison of B-mode appearance with superimposed color flow or power mode images of the residual lumen. The lesion seen in Figure 9.1 is only moderately diameter-reducing, yet this lesion produces the velocity increase that is first suspected from aliasing present at the distal portion of

Neurovascular Examination: The Rapid Evaluation of Stroke Patients Using Ultrasound Waveform Interpretation, First Edition.
Andrei V. Alexandrov.
© 2013 Andrei V. Alexandrov. Published 2013 by Blackwell Publishing Ltd.

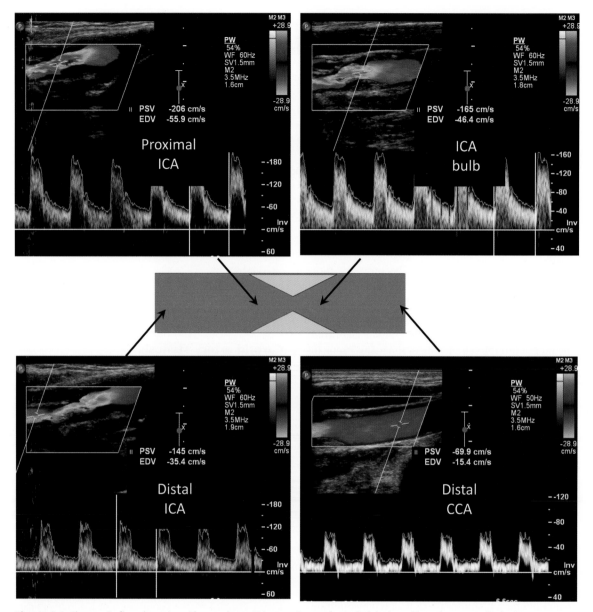

Figure 9.1 Changes in flow dynamics with a moderate ICA stenosis on color-coded duplex with angle-corrected velocity measurements. Considerations in grading the stenosis range are explained in the text.

the lesion and at the exit of the stenosis. I then look at the highest PSV value across the lesion, and calculate the highest ICA/mid-to-distal CCA velocity ratio. Figure 9.1 data show ICA PSV 206 cm/s, CCA PSV of approximately 70 cm/s, and the ratio just under 3.

I then apply the Society of Radiologists in Ultrasound (SRU) Multidisciplinary Consensus criteria

(Table 9.1) [2] and, if all measurements agree, I'm comfortable with assigning a specific range of the NASCET stenosis. It is important to emphasize the stenosis range as opposed to a specific value (i.e. 62% stenosis). Such precision is impossible to achieve [2–5] because we are using physiological data to predict how a percent diameter reduction will look on

Table 9.1 Society of Radiologists in Ultrasound (SRU) Multidisciplinary Consensus Criteria for grading focal, short, and unilateral carotid artery stenosis

Stenosis range	ICA PSV	ICA/CCA PSV ratio	ICA EDV	Plaque
Normal	<125 cm/s	<2.0	<40 cm/s	None
<50%	<125 cm/s	<2.0	<40 cm/s	<50% diameter reduction
50–69%	125–230 cm/s	2.0–4.0	40–100 cm/s	≥50% diameter reduction
70%–near occlusion	>230 cm/s	>4.0	>100 cm/s	≥50% diameter reduction
Near occlusion	May be low or undetectable	Variable	Variable	Significant, detectable lumen
Occlusion	Undetectable	Not applicable	Not applicable	Significant, no detectable lumen

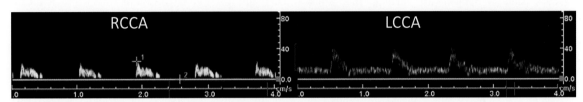

Figure 9.2 Changes in the right CCA waveform indicating high resistance to flow due to a hemodynamically significant downstream lesion (most likely an occlusion of the ICA). LCCA, left common carotid artery; RCCA, right common carotid artery.

a single-projection two-dimensional angiographic image. In this case (Figure 9.1), PSV and the ICA/CCA PSV ratio point to the 50–69% NASCET range, while B-mode suggests low–moderate plaque burden. How could these findings be reconciled? First, most plaques are axis-asymmetric and views in a longitudinal projection may not reflect the total plaque burden or the area of maximal protrusion. PSVs and the ratio are more reflective of the resulting area stenosis as well as its length, and they provide physiological information as to how the flow has adjusted to a lesion only partially seen on B-mode in any given single projection. If the PSV and the ratio findings are concordant, I often use the rule: "if two out of three measurements agree, the lesion is likely in the range predicted by these two variables." I place the weight of each measurement in descending order as follows: PSV >ICA/CCA ratio >B-mode ± flow image appearance >EDV (unless B-mode reveals a thrombus or tandem lesions).

However, the differential diagnosis in this case is not yet complete. Invasive angiography will likely underestimate the percent stenosis inherent to the choice of a single two-dimensional projection for the diameter reduction measurement and the conservative choice

of the far distal ICA as the denominator in the NASCET method. I therefore try not to over-call lesions seen on ultrasound. I would further check if the other carotid and vertebrobasilar vessels have any significant lesions. If yes, I would describe the lesion shown in Figure 9.1 as being in the 30–49% range with compensatory velocity increase. If not, I would describe it as approximately 50% stenosis caused by a mostly hypoechoic plaque of approximately 2.5 cm in length located in the ICA at origin. Factors supporting downgrading the percent stenosis (calling it closer to 50% rather then to 69%) are:

1. The CCA velocity was sampled more towards its distal portion where the velocity decreases and the actual ICA/CCA ratio could be artificially higher (i.e. closer to 3 rather then 2 where in reality it should be closer to 2 if the mid-CCA had been sampled).

2. Findings of no relative decrease in the CCA EDV, and no increase in the ICA EDV, point to a lesser degree of ICA stenosis.

As an example, look at Figure 9.2. These waveforms were obtained from the left and right CCA and there is a clear indication which vessel is now affected by an increased downstream resistance. Such a finding in the right CCA points to a severe stenosis or occlusion distal to the site of insonation, most likely in the ICA.

A word of caution: do not settle on the first and seemingly convincing findings (Figure 9.3). Figure 9.3c is a classic:

• aliasing at what appears to be the narrowest point of a stenosis caused by a hypoechoic plaque at the ICA origin/ exit from the bulb;

• Doppler waveform showing spectral "narrowing"; and

• PSV almost reaching 230 cm/s and EDV being just above 70 cm/s.

All of these findings (in one snap-shot) point to a 50–69% stenosis range, just missing the ≥70% NASCET EDV cut-off by the SRU criteria [2]. However, the rule of scanning "go with the flow" further reveals that this hypoechoic plaque is longer than just a short focal lesion seen in Figure 9.3c. Another rule – "interrogate velocities along the entire course of the lesion as long as you see the lesion" – brings you to the mid and distal parts of the ICA, fortunately traceable in this case on the neck. Findings there (though having less spectral narrowing in the mid portion) are even more convincing of the severity of the ICA stenosis: PSV increases to 298 cm/s and 490 cm/c while EDV rises to 124 cm/s and 171 cm/s respectively from the mid to distal portions. Of note, spectral narrowing reappears at the site with the PSV of 490 cm/s. The highest PSV and EDV both place the lesion in the range above 80% diameter reduction despite the appearance of a significant residual lumen on a color flow image. In a case like this, I always do a complete scan of all traceable segments along, and if possible beyond, the stenosis, and calculate the ICA/CCA PSV ratio with the highest velocity measurement (in this case the ratio has exceeded 6, images not shown). Finally, I would comment on the presence of a long (>3 cm) hypoechoic soft plaque that extends beyond the level of the jaw (remember to comment if you have or have *not* seen the distal end of the plaque as your B-mode/ flow image would be corresponding to the surgical field on the neck to expose the carotid artery).

I further use the following "rules-of-thumb" to help with grading carotid stenosis to further account if a discrepancy with the SRU criteria is found:

1. If the ICA PSV and B-mode/ color or power mode flow imaging (flow, for short) findings indicate ≥70% NASCET stenosis but ICA/CCA PSV ratio is low (i.e. <4), a compensatory velocity increase must be suspected unless CCA was sampled at its proximal portion.

2. If the ICA PSV and B-mode/ flow findings indicate ≥70% NASCET stenosis but ICA/CCA PSV ratio is very low (i.e. ≤2), a compensatory velocity increase must be suspected (there has to be a reason for collateralization of flow via this carotid artery). Remember that a contralateral lesion could be intracranial or in the vertebrobasilar system. Differential diagnosis also includes a visible unilateral CCA stenosis that could produce an artificially low ratio due to elevated CCA velocities.

3. If the ICA PSV is consistent with <70% NASCET stenosis but ICA/CCA PSV ratio and B-mode/ flow point to a severe lesion, the stenosis could be on the "other" side of the Spencer's curve [6, 7] (unless the ICA PSV was not obtained through and distal to the entire lesion [remember to visualize the distal end of the plaque and report on it] and the CCA was sampled at its distal portion).

4. If the ICA PSV, ICA/CCA PSV ratio and B-mode/ flow findings are all discrepant (i.e. PSV normal or moderately elevated, ratio is normal or significantly high, and B-mode shows a significant lesion), think about elongated (>3 cm in length stenoses), thrombi, or tandem lesions that would not produce changes predicted by the SRU criteria (which were developed for a short and unilateral ICA stenosis).

5. High PSV, high EDV, low ICA/CCA PSV ratio, and no lesion burden on B-mode/ flow usually indicate low resistance to the incoming flow (that could occur with anemia or hemodilution), and, if found particularly on one side, these findings predict either collateralization of flow, an intracranial AVM, or A–V fistulae or hyperperfusion after revascularization.

6. In the presence of a bilateral ≥50% carotid artery disease on B-mode, I use the ICA/CCA PSV ratios as the primary criterion, not necessarily the highest PSVs. The ratios help determine which side has a more severe stenosis and which one attempts to compensate for it (do not forget lesions in the posterior circulation that could also place further demand on collateralization of flow).

7. In the presence of a severe lesion on one side, I downgrade stenosis severity on the other side by one range and recommend reassessing its degree after

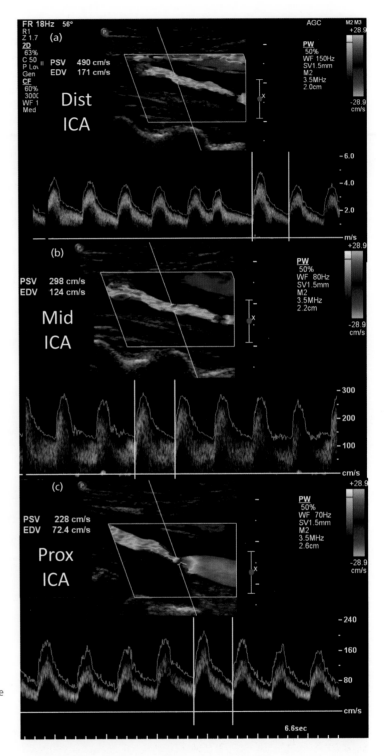

Figure 9.3 Changes in the peak systolic velocity along a hypoechoic plaque illustrate the importance of the rules: "do not settle on the first convincing image" ((**c**) proximal ICA shows spectral narrowing and the smallest residual lumen by color flow); "go with the flow" ((**a**,**b**) images demonstrate the extent of the plaque and the residual lumen); and "move Doppler sample along the entire lesion" ((**a**) the distal ICA has the highest velocities along the plaque).

revascularization of the more severe (or symptomatic) lesion.

8. If an elongated, tandem, bilateral, or "on the other side of the Spencer's curve" [7] lesion is suspected, I always perform TCD to evaluate the downstream hemodynamics and collaterals to ascertain hemodynamic significance of the proximal lesions and identify compensatory mechanisms.

In patients with symptoms of cerebral ischemia seen at our laboratory, we always perform both carotid duplex and TCD as these tests are complimentary in searching for stroke pathogenic mechanisms [8]. Even if carotid duplex interpretation is straight forward, I always look into TCD results as it may show surprises, unmasking the real hemodynamic significance of the lesion [3], distal lesion, or compensatory abilities of the circle of Willis. More on these useful findings will be discussed in the section on the downstream effects of carotid lesions.

Carotid artery occlusion

Vessel occlusions can be recent or chronic and ultrasound can detect these lesions [9]. With recent occlusions (acute or subacute), the vessel structures such as the intima–media thickness (IMT) complex are still distinguishable (Figure 9.4a). With chronic occlusion, fibrotic changes occur over time, leading to vessel collapse (Figure 9.4b), increase in lumen echogenicity, and sometimes to inability to differentiate what's left of the vessel from surrounding tissues. Further findings such as intraluminal thrombus movement, minimal pulsations transmitted with each cycle deep into the vessel with hypoechoic lumen or echogenic lumen, visible IMT, and normal-size lumen (Figure 9.5b) further support the notion that occlusion is recent (i.e. hours or days as opposed to weeks or months).

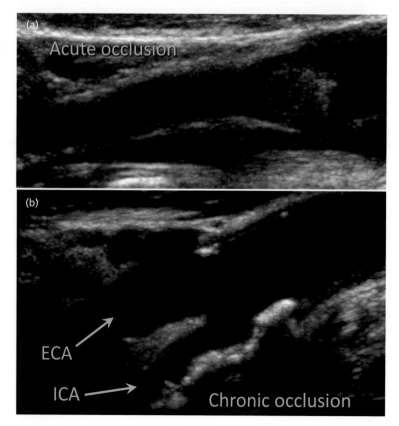

Figure 9.4 Sonographic appearances of (**a**) an acute versus (**b**) a chronic occlusion. Acute occlusion often has visible intima media complex, normal vessel lumen size, and an intraluminal thrombus. Chronic occlusion leads to vessel collapse in size, fibrosis causing increased intraluminal echogenicity, and disappearance of the intima media complex.

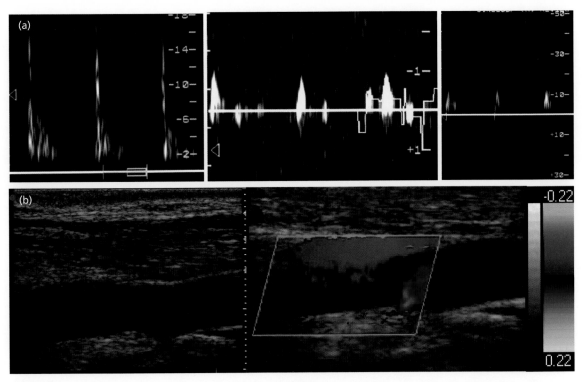

Figure 9.5 (**a**) Drum-like, systolic spike spectral waveforms and (**b**) B-mode and color flow appearance of an acute ICA thromboembolic occlusion.

What are the hallmarks of an occlusion that I look for during scanning or reviewing images? First, if an occlusion is truly complete, there should be no diastolic flow (or sometimes any flow signals) in a vessel that was supplying the brain. Color flow image can show flow void in the ICA while flow is detectable in the proximal vessel and a vein (Figure 9.5). Make sure that the angle of the color box is correct for the location of the vessel, and the color flow scale is set low as opposed to high mean Doppler shift values. Figure 9.5 shows such settings including slight over-gaining of the color box that produces a "bleeding" artifact, particularly from the venous signals. Second, if any systolic motion is detectable at the site of an occlusion, it should not be of any meaningful peak systolic velocity, nor should there be any significant trans-systolic duration of these velocities (Figure 9.5a). The next question is, what is meaningful? Systolic spikes and drum-like waveforms seen with occlusion at the ICA origin are variations of the TIBI grade 1 minimal signal [10]. Most of these waveforms have such low velocities that they could easily be eliminated by the low-frequency noise filters. So when you suspect an occlusion, reduce or even remove any spectral filters. Furthermore, even if the systolic spike reaches any significant velocity (arbitrarily 20 cm/s or more), its overall duration is usually very short, occupying a small fraction of the systolic complex. These spikes are often followed by smaller spikes, sometimes in the reversed direction, during the closure of the aortic valve (Figure 9.5a, middle image). If a sufficiently large spectral Doppler gate was deployed (that covers the entire vessel lumen), I trust those signals more. It is important to remember that gate placement near the wall in the ICA bulb with high bifurcation can mimic these signals and lead to false-positive diagnosis of an occlusion.

For confirmation of the significance of these findings, I evaluate the waveform in the feeding vessel such as the CCA. In cases with a complete ICA occlusion, the CCA diastolic flow velocity is usually greatly diminished or absent (Figure 9.2). If the CCA waveform appears normal, I suspect an occlusion that is collateralized via the reversed ophthalmic artery or a false-positive result affected by a technical error or the patient's anatomy.

Vertebral artery hypoplasia, stenosis, dissection, and occlusion

Normal vertebral arteries are often asymmetric in size, and they are usually referred to as dominant (larger) and subdominant (smaller) [11]. The difference between the subdominant and hypoplastic VA is more difficult to ascertain, as opposed to the atretic ("tiny", disappearing, or absent) VA. Further confusion arises as to when the change in caliber of the vessel occurred. Some differences could be congenital and some acquired. With our greater ability to diagnose arterial dissections, one might wonder if a proportion of what we call an accidental finding of hypoplasia or atresia developed as a result of remote dissection that did not cause a stroke, but perhaps just the neck pain. I suspect these events in patients who were athletes when they were young, or had a history of head/ neck trauma, or a motor vehicle accident in the past. Regardless, ultrasound can only help suspect hypoplasia or atresia because these conditions can only be established pathomorphologically, whereas stenosis, dissection, and complete occlusion could be better ascertained during ultrasound screening and confirmed with catheter angiography or certain MR sequences.

The main challenges in detecting, suspecting, and differentiating VA lesions are related to the following limitations of current ultrasound testing:

1. Only a limited (segmental) assessment of the VA course is attainable and short areas of a stenosis or occlusion can elude direct detection.

2. VAs can have multifocal or elongated lesions that do not produce typical abnormal findings on ultrasound and can mimic benign hypoplasia/ atresia.

3. VAs are located deep and ultrasound imaging could be inconclusive while VA origins may simply be unassessable.

Given these limitations, one should be prepared to thoroughly investigate all assessable VA segments and pay attention to waveform differences between the left and right sides, and to any waveform changes along the course of each VA.

Representative findings (Figure 9.6) of a high-resistance (PSV 41 cm/s, EDV 0 cm/s) VA waveform followed by a focal velocity jet (PSV 140 cm/s, EDV 103 cm/s) identify a severe stenosis lesion, which from an angiogram turned out to be a dissection (data not shown). Sequential findings of the absent and elevated EDV needed to be reconciled. First, absent EDV and high-resistance signals can come from a false lumen with dissection. Second, prestenotic waveforms may have minimal or no EDV if the lesion is truly severe. Furthermore, VAs can have segmental occlusions or severe stenoses that could be completely collateralized via muscular branches/ anastomoses. As a screening test, ultrasound findings in this case indicate a hemodynamically significant (i.e. severe ≥80%) VA obstruction. Such narrowing could be present with thromboembolism, atheromatous stenosis, or dissection. Consider this differential diagnosis because the intraluminal B-mode findings are suggestive of a thrombus while the high-velocity jet points to a pathological underlying process as opposed to hypoplasia or atresia that uniformly produce low-velocity/ high-resistance waveforms along the detectable course of the VA.

Systemic and cardiac abnormalities that could affect differential diagnosis

A variety of circulatory conditions affect vascular ultrasound findings and spectral waveforms [12]. The key differential algorithms that I keep in mind include the influence of the following factors on arterial waveforms:

1. variability in cardiac output, systemic vascular resistance, and blood pressure;

2. aortic valve insufficiency;

3. cardiomyopathy / congestive heart failure (CHF);

4. aortic valve stenosis;

5. atrial fibrillation.

Figure 9.7 provides schematic waveforms that could be seen with conditions 1–4.

As discussed in Chapter 8, variable cardiac output and blood pressures, particularly DBP, can produce different appearances of the diastolic complex in the waveform 1 (Figure 9.7). Deceleration of EDV could be driven by autoregulation as well as an interplay between ICP and EDV. Increased pulsatility of the

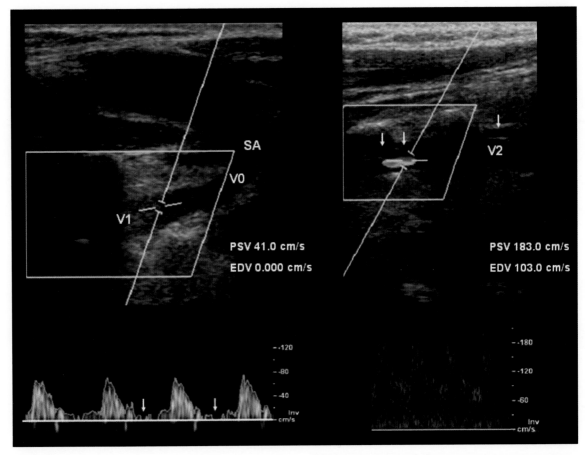

Figure 9.6 Sonographic findings with vertebral artery dissection.

waveform 1 and normal or increased EDV (dotted lines) can be a result of tachycardia or increased cardiac output.

The influence of aortic valve insufficiency is more pronounced in the proximal and extracranial vessels, while brain vasculature is able to compensate for this – an example of flow reversal negation in the MCA is shown in Figure 5.4. It is important to know about the incompetency of the valve as such waveforms may be erroneously interpreted as evidence of high resistance (i.e. elevated ICP).

Cardiomyopathy and CHF affect the ejection fraction of the heart. With patent vessels the systolic acceleration remains vertical but the systolic complex could be diminutive and such a waveform can easily be mistaken for a blunted flow signal. Hence, a low ejection fraction can lead to low velocities but compensatory cerebral vasodilation still produces a low-resistance

waveform. Velocities in these cases may never reach the values predictive of certain degrees of arterial stenoses, and parameters other then actual velocity, that is the stenotic/ prestenotic velocity ratio, needs to be used for interpretation [13].

In a case of a severe aortic valve stenosis, a delayed systolic flow acceleration should be expected in all vessels pointing to the central source of the problem. Differential diagnosis here includes Takayasu's arteritis, which could produce similar waveforms in branches distal to the affected proximal vasculature. The key is also to look at the B-mode imaging depicting arterial wall inflammation [14].

Another common condition that can affect interpretation and differentiating the degree of an arterial stenosis is atrial fibrillation (AFib). Figure 9.8 illustrates the effect of AFib on waveforms and the highest-velocity jet found with the terminal vertebral

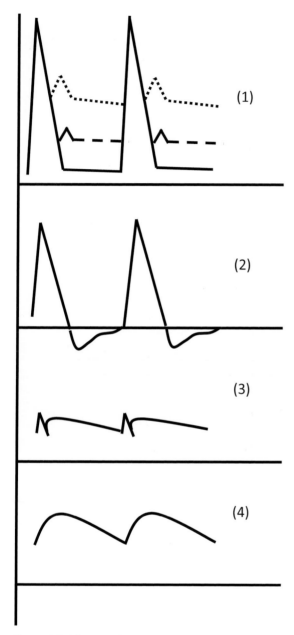

Figure 9.7 Schematic of the arterial waveforms corresponding to: (1) variable cardiac output, systemic vascular resistance, and blood pressure; (2) aortic valve insufficiency; (3) cardiomyopathy/congestive heart failure; (4) aortic valve stenosis.

artery stenosis. Although in this case AFib did not lead to underestimation of the mean flow velocity, its presence may preclude application of established velocity criteria. If velocity underestimation is a concern, other means of grading the stenosis should be used, that is ratios or downstream changes pointing to hemodynamic significance of the obstruction. In the case shown in Figure 9.8, the right vertebral artery has ≥80% stenosis as evident from a significant poststenotic turbulence in the proximal basilar artery and a blunted signal in the distal basilar artery.

Downstream effects of carotid lesions

Poststenotic or postocclusive changes observed extra- and intracranially should be used in a multiparametric assessment and grading of the severity of carotid lesions [3].

Typical findings include (Figure 9.9) [15, 16]:
1. delayed systolic flow acceleration, blunted waveforms, or tardus parvus;
2. reversed ophthalmic artery (OA);
3. recruitment of the posterior communicating artery (PComA);
4. side-to-side cross-filling via the anterior communicating artery (AComA), partial or complete;
5. indirect evidence of transcortical collateral flow recruitment;
6. decreased MCA velocities compared to the nonaffected vessels;
7. compensatory increase in collateral donor systems and vasodilation (decreased pulsatility index);
8. diminished, exhausted vasomotor reactivity [17];
9. hemodynamic steal [18];
10. microembolic signals [19].

Figure 9.9 illustrates the first seven of these effects whereas the last three are derived from additional tests that require either provocation or monitoring [17–19].

I try not to overcall the "delayed" systolic flow acceleration as this finding is not routinely measured and quantified during cerebrovascular ultrasound examinations. Instead, I rely on eye-balling and comparing the two sides or neighboring segments. Figure 9.10 shows typical delayed acceleration changes in the intracranial vessels with the proximal ICA obstruction. The MCA unilateral to an ICA obstruction is truly

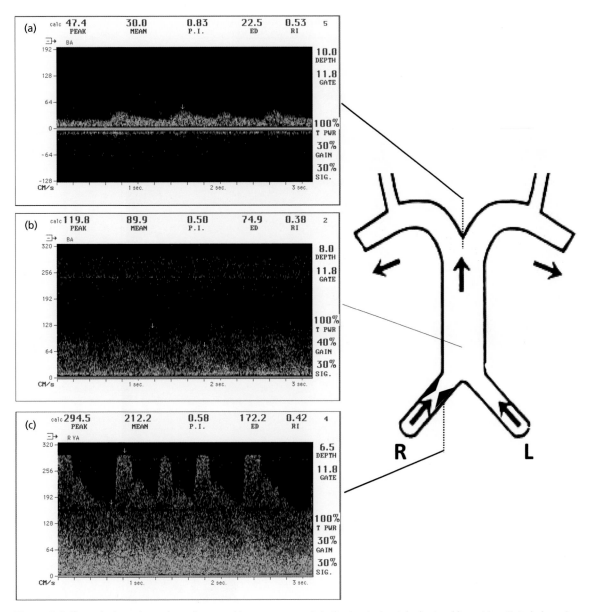

Figure 9.8 Flow velocity and waveform changes with a severe stenosis in the terminal vertebral artery (**c**); poststenotic turbulence in the proximal basilar artery (**b**); and the tardus parvus or blunted waveform in the distal basilar artery (**a**). Note that the patient also has atrial fibrillation and this irregular heart rhythm can affect automated velocity measurements. Manual cursor measurements of the single highest-velocity cardiac cycle can avoid this underestimation.

blunted; the contralateral MCA has normal systolic flow acceleration and is provided for comparison. Note a typical slight delay in systolic flow acceleration in the unobstructed posterior circulation vessels compared to the anterior circulation (contralateral MCA). This is an indirect indication of a contribution of either posterior communicating artery to the affected MCA flow or to the transcortical flow via PCA (see Figure 9.9).

The diagnosis of collaterals such as ACommA, PCommA, and reversed OA is covered in several textbooks [20–22]. The use of imaging such as transcranial duplex makes the diagnosis faster and easier [21],

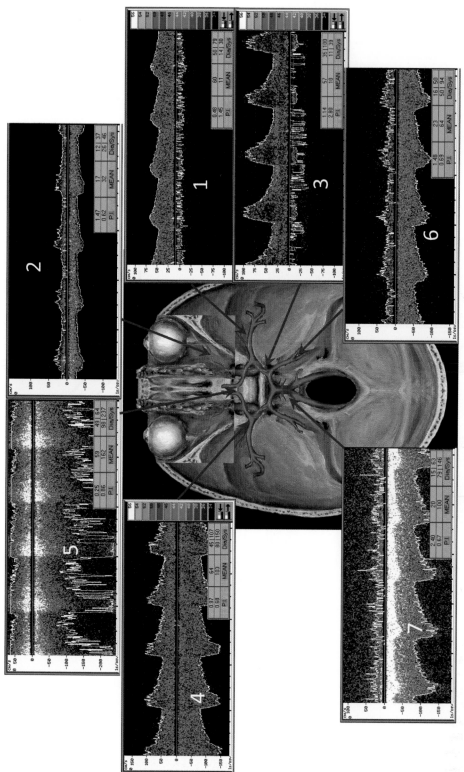

Figure 9.9 Typical intracranial waveform findings with a hemodynamically significant ICA obstruction proximal to the ophthalmic artery origin. Waveforms: (1) blunted MCA unilateral and distal to the obstructive lesion; (2) reversed ophthalmic artery; (3) posterior communicating artery waveform (note better systolic flow acceleration compared to the distal M1 MCA (waveform 1); (4) MCA above-baseline and ACA below-baseline waveforms contralateral to the ICA lesion (compensatory velocity increase MFV ACA>MCA suggesting anterior cross-filling via the anterior communicating artery); (5) stenotic velocity jet, turbulence, and bruit at the midline depth range correspond to at least partial anterior cross-filling through the anterior communicating artery; (6) compensatory velocity increase in the P2 PCA unilateral to the ICA lesion and low resistance indicate possible transcortical collateral flow; (7) double waveform at the junction of the vertebral arteries and the proximal basilar artery with compensatory velocity increase in the dominant vertebral/ proximal basilar artery.

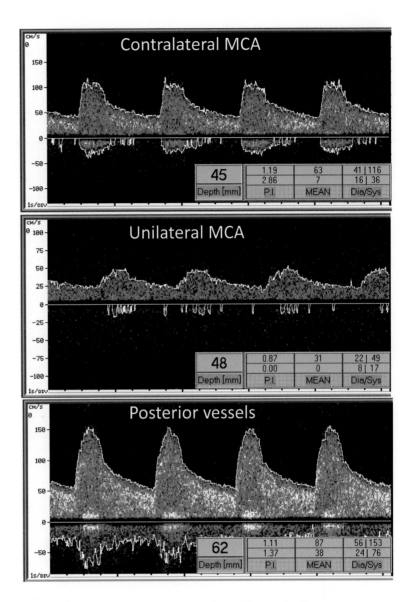

Figure 9.10 Typical intracranial waveforms with a proximal ICA obstruction. Note differences in the systolic flow acceleration between the MCA on the affected and nonaffected sides, and between the anterior and posterior circulation vessels. These changes help differentiate waveform origins without image-guided duplex sonography.

particularly for the PCommA. In suspecting and identifying main collaterals such as ACommA and PCommA, the closer the ultrasound study is performed to symptom onset or the acute progression of an obstruction, the more obvious the velocity changes are. For example, the donor side MCA/ACA or PCA/BA have higher velocities than the recipient MCA. Next, the MCA unilateral to the carotid lesion has higher velocity the more proximal it is to the supporting collateral channel. It is very important to see continuity of these signals and not to rely on limited or partial examinations. The next section will describe

the aspects of the differential diagnosis between intracranial stenoses and collaterals.

An intracranial hemodynamic steal and its impact on vasomotor reactivity will be discussed in a subsequent chapter. While performing and storing ultrasound test results, the sonographer should pay close attention also to the presence of spontaneous artery-to-artery embolization, which sometimes is the only sign of a partial and nonhemodynamically significant obstruction by an embolus to the ICA or a thrombus over an ulcerated plaque surface. These multiple findings should be considered in determination of the range of the ICA stenosis as well as its location relative to carotid duplex findings on the neck [3].

Intracranial stenoses versus collaterals

One of the main issues leading to the difficulty identifying stenosis versus collateralization of flow is the fact that the velocity does not equate to flow volume [23]. In other words, a high-velocity jet may reflect a decreased, normal, or increased flow volume. This is true with carotid duplex imaging findings on the neck, and this is also true for transcranial Doppler examinations. To help differentiate changes in flow volume, various ratios for assessment of the degree of arterial narrowing can be used as they qualitatively reflect increased or decreased flow volume states:
1. ICA/CCA PSV ratio (carotid duplex) (≤2.0 and ≥4.0 respectively) [2];
2. stenotic/ prestenotic intracranial vessel ratios (TCD/ TCCS) (≤2.0 and ≥3.0) [13];
3. Lindegaard/ Soustiel ratios (TCD in SAH) (<3 and ≥6; ≤2.0 and ≥3.0) [24–26].

Besides these dichotomized values, one can also look at any actual ratio value and consider whether it corresponds to the velocity. As an example, if the Lindegaard ratio is 4.1 but the MCA MFV is 210 cm/s, this finding may not indicate a severe vasospasm but rather moderate spasm with some hyperemia (or a hyperdynamic component).

Regardless of the specific location (extra- or intracranial) or the presence of certain pathologies (carotid disease, intracranial stenoses, or vasospasm/ hyperemia considerations), I determine the following to decide if the velocity increase is due to an obstruction or if it is compensatory:
1. Is there any evidence for a structural lesion? This could be direct imaging findings of a plaque, thrombus, or aliasing on color flow at the intracranial focal flow jet narrowing.
2. If there is such evidence, is the lesion focal (short or long), tandem, or diffuse? Length of a plaque, stenosis location, discovery of presumed poststenotic flow signals, or spasm location could provide clues.
3. Is the lesion of the up-slope or on the other side of the Spencer's curve [7]? This will provide information if the velocity increase and the corresponding ratio are trustworthy or the ratio is giving a more accurate assessment than the velocity.
4. Is there a need for collateral flow? The presence of a contralateral lesion or a proximal or distal unilateral lesion could create the demand.
5. Could both a stenosis and collateral flow (or spasm and a hyperdynamic state) be present across the insonated segment?

If one sets out to detect intracranial atherosclerotic disease (IAD), there are fairly straightforward criteria to find focal significant MFV increases predictive of ≥50% and ≥70% stenoses or paradoxical velocity decreases with very severe lesions/ near occlusions, or diffuse intracranial disease (Table 9.2) [13].

If one encounters difficulty differentiating downstream effects of the carotid lesions and potential involvement of the ACommA or PCommA, location of high-velocity jets will be more telling about collaterals. In Figure 9.9, ACommA high-velocity jet is found at depths of 70–80 mm (midline) with anterior angulation of the probe. Using transcranial duplex imaging can aid greatly the vessel identification [21].

Table 9.2 Our neurovascular ultrasound laboratory criteria for grading intracranial atherosclerotic disease (IAD)

Stenosis range	MFV MCA	SPR	MFV VB	SPR
Normal	<80 cm/s	<2	<60 cm/s	<2
<50%	<100 cm/s	<2	<90 cm/s	<2
≥50%	≥100 cm/s	≥2	≥90 cm/s	≥2
≥70%	≥120 cm/s	≥3	≥110 cm/s	≥3
Diffuse IAD or near occlusion	<30 cm/s	<1	<20 cm/s	<1

SPR, stenotic/ prestenotic MFV ratio; VB, vertebrobasilar arteries.

Of particular interest are cases when collateralization of flow is induced in the posterior circulation vessels by the presence of an ICA lesion. One or both vertebral arteries start to carry collateral flow that is then directed through the basilar towards the posterior communicating artery or the PCA, if the transcortical collateralization of flow is also involved. Yet, the vertebral arteries or the basilar artery may have additional stenoses, or the vertebral arteries may have congenital endings in the posterior inferior cerebellar artery (PICA), or that often-hypoplastic segment and PICA may now need to transport collateral flow if another vertebral is chronically occluded. Figure 9.11 provides examples of the waveforms in both terminal

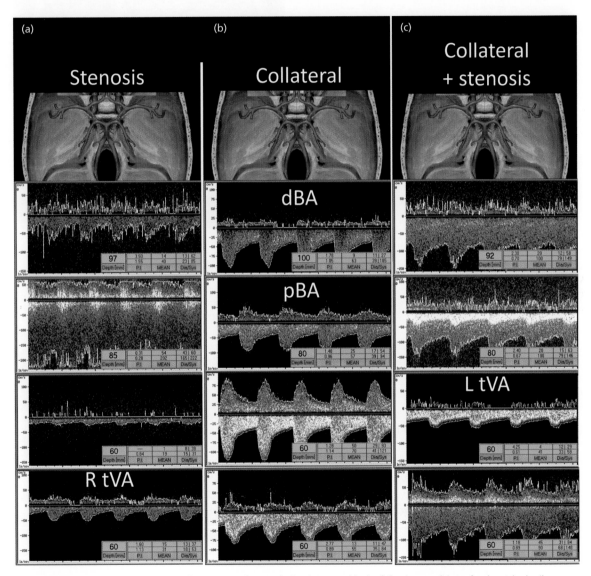

Figure 9.11 Three case examples that illustrate waveform/ velocity changes with the following conditions: focal vertebrobasilar stenosis/ no collateralization/ no ICA lesion (**a**); collateralization due to an ICA lesion and no focal vertebrabasilar stenosis (**b**); vertebrobasilar stenosis and collateralization of flow due to an ICA lesion (**c**). Depth of insonation and velocity/ pulsatility data are provided in inserts for each waveform. Each row of waveforms across all columns corresponds to (from bottom to the top): right terminal vertebral artery (R tVA); left terminal vertebral artery (L tVA); proximal basilar artery (pBA); and distal basilar artery (dBA).

vertebral, proximal, and distal basilar arteries in three cases: focal VB stenosis/ no collateralization/ no ICA lesion; collateralization/ ICA lesion/ no focal VB stenosis; VB stenosis/ collateralization/ ICA lesion.

Intracranial occlusion localization

The majority of acute intracranial occlusions that are detectable with current imaging methods, including catheter angiography, are located at the following levels of the vasculature:

1. cortical branches (third, or sometimes even further levels subdivisions);

2. second-degree subdivisions (i.e. M2, A2, P2, or main trunks of the cerebellar arteries);

3. main stems (M1, A1, P1, basilar artery);

4. terminal portions of the arteries entering the skull (terminal ICAs and VAs);

5. proximal vessels (ICA, CCA, VA);

6. tandem or multiple lesions.

The accuracy of our ability to detect these lesions increases with the more proximal location of the obstruction and with its greater hemodynamic significance (i.e. complete vs. partial as well as major proximal vessel vs. distal branch). Figure 9.12 illustrates proximal occlusion locations directly or indirectly detectable by transcranial ultrasound. The following will demonstrate which findings, in addition to the TIBI residual flow grading system [10], I look for to differentiate the level of obstruction and the presence of tandem lesions.

How to differentiate occlusion location?

(reproduced with permission, © Health Outcomes Institute, Inc. 2011)

This algorithm is based on accounting for hemodynamic significance or flow disturbances of an acute arterial obstruction at any proximal and detectable level. These acute lesions can also invoke compensatory mechanisms such as flow diversion and collateralization. These findings should also be put together with progressive decrease in the residual flow grade from proximal to distal segments (i.e. TIBI 5(±4), 3, 2, 1, and 0 as one advances insonation from feeding and proximal vessels to the distal and more affected parts). For simplicity, the depth of the worst residual flow

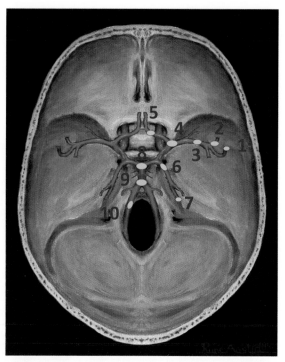

Figure 9.12 Occlusion locations directly or indirectly detectable by transcranial ultrasound. The circle of Willis drawing (courtesy of Dr Rune Aaslid) was modified. Locations: (1) distal M2/M3 MCA (high resistance in the feeding vessel and signs of flow diversion to another branch or ACA or PCA); (2) proximal M2 MCA (abnormal TIBI waveform or high resistance in the proximal vessels and flow diversion); (3) M1 MCA (abnormal TIBI waveform and flow diversion); (4) terminal ICA (abnormal TIBI waveform and signs of collateralization of flow in the contralateral anterior circulation or unilateral posterior circulation vessels; often stenotic signals found at depths 65 mm or greater); (5) A1 ACA (abnormal TIBI waveform and possible flow diversion); (6) P1 PCA (abnormal TIBI waveform and possible flow diversion); (7) P2 PCA (abnormal TIBI waveform or high resistance in the feeding segment and possible flow diversion); (8) top-of-the-basilar (abnormal TIBI waveform and signs of flow diversion to the anterior circulation vessels and proximal cerebellar arteries); (9) proximal basilar artery (abnormal TIBI waveform and flow diversion); (10) terminal vertebral artery (abnormal TIBI waveform and flow diversion). Detailed explanations of criteria and differential algorithm are provided in the text.

signal is equated with the occlusion location. In reality, partial obstruction and thrombus length may further contribute to the hemodynamic significance of the lesion and thus help in localization of an acute occlusion. The algorithm includes the following steps:

1. Identify the worst residual TIBI flow grade.

2. Depth of the worst residual flow reflects the following:

   (a) ≤30 mm distal M2/cortical branches (temporal window)

   (b) 30–40 mm M2 MCA (temporal window)

   (c) 40–65 mm M1 MCA (temporal window), 40–80 mm terminal VA (foraminal window)

   (d) 60–70 mm terminal ICA (temporal window)

   (e) 60–80 mm A1 ACA (temporal window)

   (f) 80–120 mm contralateral terminal ICA/ M1 MCA (temporal window) 80–110 mm basilar artery (foraminal window).

3. Remember that TIBI 1, 2, and 3 signals can be found at shallow (<40 mm) depths due to the presence of numerous vessels at close to 90 degree interception angles. TIBI 0 signal can be due to the ultrasound beam not intercepting a vessel or no bony window. Therefore, to locate branch occlusion one must find supportive evidence:

   (a) Flow diversion to a neighboring branch (normal of high-velocity, positive diastolic flow, the involved branch PI is less than PI in a nonaffected; homologous segment if the velocity is equal or lower to the normal side)

   (b) Presence of a detectable normal flow signal at a similar depth range on the nonaffected side.

4. No specific criteria exist for TCD to identify the cerebellar branch occlusions.

5. If TIBI 0–3 waveforms are found at 40–65 mm depths (temporal window) or 40–80 mm (foraminal window), find flow diversion to the first segment unilateral branches, i.e. A1 ACA, P1 PCA for MCA lesions, or contralateral VA, uni- or contralateral PICA for tVA/proximal BA lesions.

6. If no flow diversion exists, confirm the asymmetry of flow velocities with the nonaffected vessel (MCA) or patent terminal vertebral artery (tVA) (VA or proximal BA occlusions). The affected side should have at least 30% MFV reduction or absent diastolic flow. The greater the asymmetry between the homologous segments, the greater the likelihood of true positive findings of an occlusion.

7. If abnormal TIBI flow signals are found at the depth ranges of the terminal ICA of the basilar artery, confirm the presence of collateralization of flow either through the contralateral ICA and VB system (TICA occlusions) or ICA(s) or at in least one VA/PICA (BA occlusion).

8. If a stenotic signal is found at midline depths (70–80 mm) or the nonaffected TICA/MCA/ACA have the velocity increase above age expected values with low pulsatility of flow, these findings are indicative of the ICA, TICA, or BA occlusions. Differential includes pre-existing intracranial stenosis. Findings of ACommA (complete or partial cross-filling) or PCommA or transcrotical flow unmask those proximal lesions.

9. The presence of embolic signals in the vessels affected by ischemia indicates a proximal source that could be an unstable plaque, artery-to-artery embolization in the setting of atherothrombosis, or partially occlusive embolus in the feeding vessel.

10. Blunted or extremely flattened low-velocity signal in the MCA traceable from 65 mm to 30 mm implies the presence of an ICA or TICA obstruction with poor collateralization of flow via circle of Willis. Similar tenuous flow in the basilar artery at depths 80–100 mm implies the dominant terminal vertebral/ proximal basilar obstruction with lack of efficient cross-cerebellar or reversed top-of-the basilar collateralization of flow.

11. TIBI 0, 1, or 2 in the MCA and collateralization of flow via ACommA, PCommA, or transcortical flow imply the presence of a tandem MCA/TICA or MCA/ICA lesion.

12. Absent flow signals through the entire anterior circulation depths imply no window (rule out by locating PCA flow or contralateral vessels over the same window), or no flow with TICA occlusion. TICA occlusion could be of L-type (TICA/MCA occlusion), T-type (TICA/MCA/ACA), or the anterior trifurcation type (TICA/MCA/ACA/PCA) with the so-called "fetal" origin of the PCA:

   (a) L-type will have abnormal TIBI signals at 30–70 mm depths plus stenotic signals at midline or contralateral MFV ACA>MCA, or unilateral PCommA, or transcortical collateral flow findings;

   (b) T-type will have partial anterior cross-filling or PCommA or transcortical collateral flow findings;

(c) Anterior trifurcation TICA occlusion could either have no detectable signals over the entire unilateral temporal window, or abnormal TIBI signals in both anterior and posterior circulation vessels and the presence of partial anterior cross-filling via ACommA.

13. Top of the basilar occlusion may have abnormal TIBI signals located at ≥100 mm depth through the foraminal window and at 70–80 mm depths through the temporal window with perpendicular or slightly posterior angulation of the probe via the midtemporal or posterior aspect of the temporal window. This occlusion location can be accompanied by flow diversion to PICA and other cerebellar arteries as well as ICA(s) and MCA(s) with signs of recruitment anterior-to-posterior collateral flow.

14. Isolated P1 or P2 PCA occlusions can be found at 55–75 mm depths via the temporal window and may not be accompanied by detectable flow diversion signs as these vessels carry the least amount of flow volume and have limited transcortical collateralization capacities that may not affect flow parameters at M1 A1 and M2 vessel levels. In addition, remember that hypoplasia of P1 PCA is common.

15. Tandem VB lesions may be found with a variety of abnormal TIBI flow signals at various depths through the foraminal and temporal windows for P1 and P2 PCAs. These findings should be differentiated from chronic conditions, tortuosity, and suboptimal insonation angles through findings of collateralization of flow to cerebellar vessels, retrograde filling of the basilar artery, and flow diversion/ collateralization through the anterior circulation vessels.

16. Retrograde basilar artery flow can be found at depths 80–100 mm towards the probe and with abnormal antergrade TIBI flow signals at the level of the terminal vertebral arteries and the basilar artery.

Typical occlusion locations, waveforms, and correlative imaging can also be found in *Cerebrovascular Ultrasound in Diagnosis and Management* [20], which has a chapter on the diagnostic criteria for cerebrovascular ultrasound, and also in other parts of this book.

Vasospasm

Detection, grading, and monitoring vasospasm after subarachnoid hemorrhage has been the first clinical application for TCD [27]. This was developed by Rune Aaslid so that neurosurgeons and intensivists do not have to "fly in the dark" regarding which patients are developing vasospasm and which will have a severe spasm that will likely lead to a delayed neurological deficit secondary to ischemia, which the untreated vasospasm can produce.

Over the past 30 years, numerous studies have shown that TCD is a moderate-to-good predictor of the proximal vasospasm [28]. The original MFV and Lindegaard ratio criteria for vasospasm were conceptualized in the 1980s, and since then neurocritical care for these patients has evolved as well as pharmacological management. Thus, traditional TCD criteria came under scrutiny [29], and now is the time to revisit these criteria and perhaps adjust for age, and therapies that are vasoactive or affect hemorheology. In the absence of such new validation studies, I use the following velocity/ ratio criteria (Tables 9.3, 9.4, and 9.5) and algorithm to detect vasospasm and point to possible contribution of hyperdynamic states.

1. Determine baseline MFV for each individual patient for each vessel. Even though most adults will have normal velocities below 120 cm/s, age-specific data are not yet in wide use, and each patient could serve as their own control to evaluate the dynamics over time in each detectable intracranial vessel.

2. Sample MFV in 12 key intracranial segments: (distal MCA, proximal MCA, A1 ACA, PCA) × 2 plus two VAs, proximal and distal BA [30].

3. Obtain data daily for comparison: baseline <48 hours from Day 0, daily for Days 3–7 to detect which patient is developing vasospasm.

4. I use the following MFV thresholds: MCA ≥ 120 cm/s, ACA ≥ 110 cm/s, TICA ≥ 90 cm/s. PCA, BA, VA ≥ 70 cm/s for the presence of any vasospasm (Sloan's criteria) [31, 32].

5. If baseline MFV was higher than age-expected (i.e. MFV >65 cm/s in a patient older than 65 years, or MFV >100 cm/s in a patient less than 45 years of age), and the diagnostic angiogram within 48 hours from Day 0 did not show any spasm, I use "double the initial velocity" rule to determine if a patient is developing any vasospasm in the future.

6. Even though in the first 5 days I use the most sensitive criteria to detect any spasm development, I'm also checking for any vasoactive or hemodilut-

Table 9.3 TCD criteria for grading the proximal MCA vasospasm*

Mean flow velocity (cm/s)	MCA/ICA MFV ratio	Interpretation
<120	≤3	Normal
≥120	3–4	Development of mild spasm + hyperemia
≥120	4–5	Moderate spasm + hyperemia
>120	5–6	Moderate spasm
≥180	6	Moderate-to-severe spasm
≥200	≥6	Severe spasm
>200	4–6	Moderate spasm + hyperemia
>200	3–4	Hyperemia + mild (often residual) spasm
>200	<3	Hyperemia

*Note that listed velocity cut-offs are applicable to patients whose baseline MFVs (before vasospasm) were below 60 cm/s. If MFVs are >60 cm/s on Days 0–2, I use double and triple the baseline MFV values to identify the beginning and progression of vasospasm instead of 120 and 200 cm/s thesholds. Further velocity corrections are needed to individually adjust for age, hematocrit, and vasoactive/ hemodilution treatments.

Table 9.4 Sloan's optimized criteria for grading vasospasm in the intracranial arteries [31, 32]

Artery	MFV (cm/s)		
	Possible VSP*	Probable VSP*	Definite VSP*
ICA	>80	>110	>130
ACA	>90	>110	>120
PCA	>60	>80	>90
BA	>70	>90	>100
VA	>60	>80	>90

*After hyperemia has been mostly ruled out by the focal velocity increase and by the intracranial artery/ extracranial ICA ratio ≥3 except for posterior circulation vessels.

ing treatment the patient may receive. These treatments can elevate MFV artificially thus making any single MFV value less predictive of the degree of vasospasm.

7. Once abnormal elevation of MFV is found, I do not call any significance of vasospasm until Lindegaard ratio exceeds 3 or Soustiel ratio exceeds 2. Even though the original research with these ratios found that these values are predictive of moderate vasospasm, the fact remains that catheter angiography is a more conservative way of determining spasm severity.

8. I monitor daily dynamics of abnormal MFVs and extend daily monitoring to Day 10, and if MFVs remain abnormal, I monitor until Day 14.

9. During this time interval, I look for MFV ≥200 cm/s for MCA or Lindegaard ratio of ≥6 to identify patients with severe vasospasm. In fact, I rely more on the ratio, provided that the submandibular ICA sampling has been consistent for its calculation.

10. I grade other vessels by at least a threefold increase from the baseline velocity or reference vessel to identify severe stages of vasospasm.

11. I expect that most patients will be developing vasospasm in one of these four locations:

    (a) MCA/TICA + ACA;

    (b) bilateral A1 ACA;

    (c) terminal VA/basilar artery vasospasm;

    (d) distal branches.

12. Upon resolution (intervention, time course, etc.), I look for decreasing Linegaard or Soustiel ratios in the first place as in some patients velocities may remain high for several reasons (persistence of spasm with good compensation, concurrent hemodilution, or infection).

13. In a small number of patients, late recurrent vasospasm can occur or persistence of severe spasm can cause focal neurological symptoms beyond Days

Table 9.5 Sviri's optimized criteria for grading vasospasm in the basilar artery using Soustiel's ratio [25, 26]

Vasospasm	Soustiel's ratio*	BA MFV velocity	Sensitivity	Specificity
BA vasospasm	>2	>70 cm/s	77%	82%
Moderate or severe BA vasospasm	>2.5	>85 cm/s	86%	97%
Severe BA vasospasm	>3	>85 cm/s	92%	97%

*Soustiel's ratio: MFV BA/MFV EXVA. MFV, mean flow velocity; BA, basilar artery; EXVA, extracranial vertebral artery sampled at the first cervical level, depth 45–55 mm.

10–12, and in these patients I monitor ratio dynamics, particularly when hypertension or hemodilution portions of medical management are de-escalating in patients with persistently elevated velocities.

Of all spasm locations, distal branches are the most elusive for TCD. It can be missed completely, or found indirectly when it is already hemodynamically significant and causes flow diversion via proximal branches. These findings may already be too late for timely intervention.

Therefore, the best way to practice TCD surveillance of vasospasm is to provide daily diagnostic studies every morning at the time of, or prior to, neurosurgery/ neurocritical care team rounds, and repeat studies during the day or urgently if certain vasoactive medication adjustments are made or neurological changes are noticed in a patient.

Hyperemia

Hyperemia in cerebrovascular ultrasound literature is a broad term that is often used to qualitatively describe an increased blood flow volume or perfusion based on velocity/ pulsatility changes rather than actual blood flow volume measurements. It is common after SAH (differential with vasospasm and its relative contribution are discussed above and shown in Table 9.3). This term is also used in stroke management as it may occur after carotid revascularization [33], systemic tPA treatment, and intra-arterial reperfusion [34].

Hyperemia should be on the differential diagnosis list when elevated velocities and low PI values are found in the intracranial, and sometimes feeding extracranial, vessels. A combination of a stenosis and hyperdynamic states may also exist. Clinically, patients with postrevascularization hyperemia frequently experience headache and seizures (i.e. hyperperfusion syndrome). TCD findings of ≥50% absolute increase in MFV compared to preprocedure values in the MCA unilateral to a reconstructed carotid artery and low-pulsatility waveforms compared to the contralateral side point to hyperemia or hyperperfusion.

Lower resistance to flow compared to the contralateral side indicates a decreased capacity of the distal vasculature to regulate the re-established flow volume under current blood pressure values. Pulsatility index decrease by >20% compared to the contralateral side serves as additional indicator. Because PI is quite variable and could be affected by multiple factors, make sure that both sides were studied at rest or in a steady state position and without the patient talking, performing tasks, or hyperventilating.

These changes can be found during surgery immediately after ICA cross-clamp release [33]. Hyperperfusion should be suspected if the MCA MFV becomes 1.5 times the pre-cross-clamp values and persists at that level without corrective measures for 2 minutes or more [33].

Hyperemic reperfusion can also be observed with systemic thrombolytic therapy and intra-arterial revascularization procedures for acute ischemic stroke [34]. These findings may precede hemorrhagic transformation and may require even tighter blood pressure control to avoid complications of reperfusion. Figure 9.13 shows examples of nonhyperemic recanalization distal to a persisting proximal ICA occlusion (Figure 9.13a) and hyperemic reperfusion on an isolated M1 MCA occlusion (Figure 9.13b) that resulted

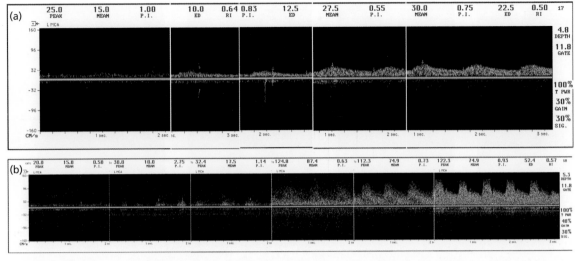

Figure 9.13 Examples of nonhyperemic (**a**) and hyperemic (**b**) complete MCA recanalization during systemic tPA therapy. The upper images show recanalization of the MCA to MFV >20cm/s and blunted waveform due to persisting proximal ICA occlusion. The images in (**b**) indicate complete MCA recanalization to TIBI 5 flow with elevated MFV relative to the patient's age and low resistance.

in a fatal hemorrhagic transformation. Our preliminary criteria for differentiating hyperemic reperfusion from TIBI 4 flow after acute reperfusion therapies for stroke are:

1. uniform post initial recanalization velocity elevation along the course of the proximal vessel of >30% compared to the nonaffected homologous vessel segment;

2. PI is lower compared to the nonaffected vessel by >20%;

3. absence of distal obstruction to flow as determined from lack of abnormal TIBI flow grades, indicating persisting obstruction, and flow velocity decrease in the proximal branching vessels, indicating cessation of flow diversion.

Of note, some flow diversion may continue to exist particularly if hyperemic reperfusion affects only one major branch that recanalized while the other one remains obstructed. Therefore, it is important to continue to survey the branches for persistence of a distal occlusion.

Steal

The concept of an arterial blood flow steal has been applied to coronary [35], extracranial [36], and intrac-

ranial vessels [37] to explain hemodynamic changes with acute occlusions, subclavian artery stenoses (Figure 9.14), and arteriovenous malformations and fistulas. We are now able to detect and quantify arterial steal in patients with cerebral ischemia [37].

The hallmark of a steal is flow diversion. It can manifest as:

1. a compensatory velocity increase in the donor vessel due to recruitment of collaterals by vasodilation in tissues with compromised perfusion (natural steal by vessels distal to an arterial occlusion [35], i.e. "rob the rich to feed the poor"), or

2. changes in flow direction during the cardiac cycle (in case of a subclavian steal present at rest or invoked by transient hyperemia; Figure 9.14), or by

3. paradoxical velocity behavior in response to vasodilatory stimuli (velocity decrease in the affected vessels simultaneously with an increase observed in the normal vasculature, i.e. "rob the poor to feed the rich", or the "reversed" Robin Hood principle) [37].

Thus, a collateral channel can act as a double-edge sword, that is delivering sufficient supplies under favorable circulatory conditions and depriving tissues at risk of supply when the pressure gradient favors normally perfused tissues.

Steals can occur at any level of circulation. Proximal intracranial vessels are better targets as our current

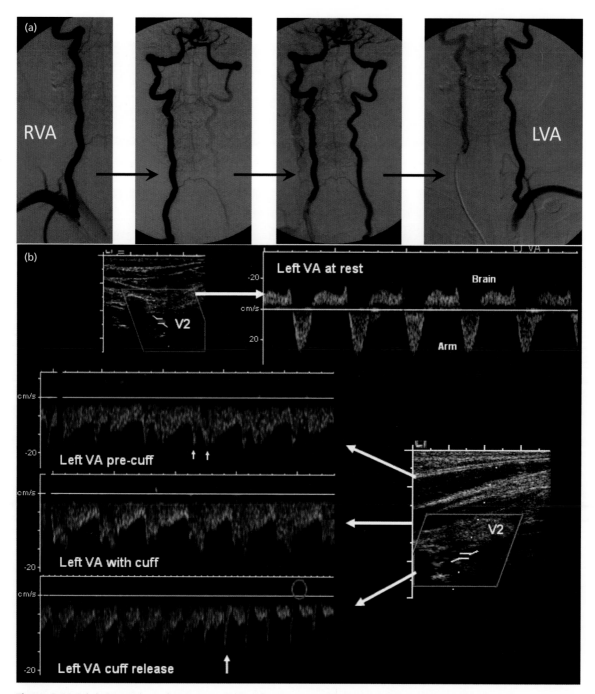

Figure 9.14 Subclavian steal waveforms at rest and with hyperemia test (**b**). Catheter angiograms (**a**) shows the steal on sequential frames (from the right vertebral artery injection contrast goes to the reversed or stealing left vertebral artery).

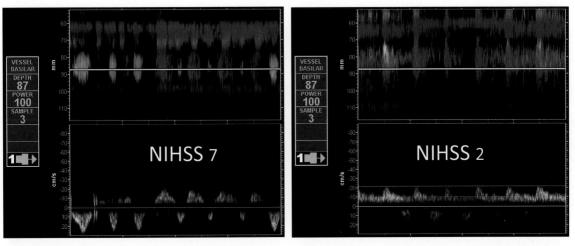

Figure 9.15 Case example of symptomatic steal in the basilar artery due to insufficient cardiac function producing neurological symptoms/ worsening and its correction with pressors. Time-corresponding National Institutes of Health Stroke Scale (NIHSS) scores are provided for each waveform.

tools are more capable of sampling these vessels. As technology develops, smaller branches and arterioles could be studied and the frequency of steal detection should increase. The following case demonstrates steal occurrence in a focal area of the posterior circulation leading to the reversed Robin Hood syndrome [37].

A 75-year-old man with known CHF presented to ER with shortness of breath and diaphoresis. He subsequently developed slurred speech along with fluctuating and decreasing level of consciousness. Figure 9.15 shows the diastolic flow reversal on TCD in the terminal vertebral as well as the proximal and midbasilar artery (depth range 76–95 mm). His BP was 92/70 mmHg at that time and his NIHSS was 7. Dobutamine 2 mg infusion was started, his BP increased to 105/74, TCD showed reappearance of the positive EDV at these depths, and his NIHSS decreased to 2 points. His NIHSS was 0 after 2 hours of dobutamine infusion and he was evaluated for continuing treatment with an intra-aortic balloon pump.

To diagnose steal and differentiate it from other causes, it is important to maintain a steady angle of insonation and have the system challenged with one stimulus at a time. Ideally, a proximal branching point with vessels supplying both affected and nonaffected vasculature should be sampled simultaneously. Alternatively, postobstructive flow and a homologous con-tralateral segment should be sampled at the same time and velocity behavior should be evaluated simultaneously in response to naturally occurring or induced stimulus.

References

1. Alexandrov AV, Needleman L. Carotid artery stenosis: making complex assessments of a simple problem or simplifying approach to a complex disease? *Stroke* 2012; **43**: 627–8.
2. Grant EG, Benson, CB, Moneta, GL, *et al.* Carotid artery stenosis: gray-scale and Doppler US diagnosis – Society of Radiologists in Ultrasound Consensus Conference. *Radiology* 2003; **229**: 340–6.
3. von Reutern GM, Goertler MW, Bornstein NM, *et al*; Neurosonology Research Group of the World Federation of Neurology. Grading carotid stenosis using ultrasonic methods. *Stroke* 2012; **43**: 916–21.
4. Toole JF, Castaldo JE. Accurate measurement of carotid stenosis. Chaos in methodology. *J Neuroimaging* 1994; **4**: 222–30.
5. Faught WE, Mattos MA, van Bemmelen PS, *et al.* Color-flow duplex scanning of carotid arteries: new velocity criteria based on receiver operator characteristic analysis for threshold stenoses used in the symptomatic and asymptomatic carotid trials. *J Vasc Surg* 1994; **19**: 818–27.

6. Spencer MP, Reid JM. Quantitation of carotid stenosis with continuous wave Doppler ultrasound. *Stroke* 1979; **10**: 326–30.

7. Alexandrov AV. The Spencer's curve: clinical implications of a classic hemodynamic model. *J Neuroimaging* 2007; **17**: 6–10.

8. Alexandrov AV, Sloan MA, Tegeler CH, *et al*; for the American Society of Neuroimaging Practice Guidelines Committee. Practice standards for transcranial Doppler (TCD) ultrasound. Part II. Clinical indications and expected outcomes. *J Neuroimaging* 2012; **22**: 215–24.

9. Blackshear WM Jr, Phillips DJ, Thiele BL, *et al*. Detection of carotid occlusive disease by ultrasonic imaging and pulsed Doppler spectrum analysis. *Surgery* 1979; **86**: 698–706.

10. Demchuk AM, Burgin WS, Christou I, *et al*. Thrombolysis in Brain Ischemia (TIBI) transcranial Doppler flow grades predict clinical severity, early recovery, and mortality in patients treated with tissue plasminogen activator. *Stroke* 2001; **32**: 89–93.

11. George B, Bruneau M, Spetzler RF (eds). *Pathology and Surgery Around the Vertebral Artery*. Vienna: Springer, 2011.

12. Bendick PJ. Cardiac effects on peripheral arterial waveforms. *J Vasc Ultrasound* 2011; **35**: 237–43.

13. Zhao L, Barlinn K, Sharma VK, *et al*. Velocity criteria for intracranial stenosis revisited: an international multicenter study of transcranial Doppler and digital subtraction angiography. *Stroke* 2011; **42**: 3429–34.

14. Sun Y, Yip PK, Jeng JS, *et al*. Ultrasonographic study and long-term follow-up of Takayasu's arteritis. *Stroke* 1996; **27**: 2178–82.

15. Wilterdink JL, Feldmann E, Furie KL, *et al*. Transcranial Doppler ultrasound battery reliably identifies severe internal carotid artery stenosis. *Stroke* 1997; **28**: 133–6.

16. Christou I, Felberg RA, Demchuk AM, *et al*. Accuracy parameters of a broad diagnostic battery for bedside transcranial Doppler to detect flow changes with internal carotid artery stenosis or occlusion. *J Neuroimaging* 2001; **11**: 236–42.

17. Ringelstein EB, Weiller C, Weckesser M, *et al*. Cerebral vasomotor reactivity is significantly reduced in low-flow as compared to thromboembolic infarctions: the key role of the circle of Willis. *J Neurol Sci* 1994; **121**: 103–9.

18. Alexandrov AV, Sharma VK, Lao AY, *et al*. Reversed Robin Hood syndrome in acute ischemic stroke patients. *Stroke* 2007; **38**: 3045–8.

19. Markus HS, King A, Shipley M, *et al*. Asymptomatic embolisation for prediction of stroke in the Asymptomatic Carotid Emboli Study (ACES): a prospective observational study. *Lancet Neurol* 2010; **9**: 663–71.

20. Alexandrov AV. *Cerebrovascular Ultrasound in Stroke Prevention and Treatment*, 2nd edn. Oxford: Wiley-Blackwell Publishers, 2011.

21. Valdueza JM, Shreiber SJ, Roehl JE, *et al. Neurosonology and Neuroimaging of Stroke*. Stuttgart: Georg Thieme Verlag, 2008.

22. von Reutern GM, Budingen HJ. *Ultrasound Diagnosis of Cerebrovascular Disease*. Stuttgart: Georg Thieme Verlag, 1993.

23. Kontos HA. Validity of cerebral arterial blood flow calculations from velocity measurements. *Stroke* 1989; **20**: 1–3.

24. Lindegaard KF. The role of transcranial Doppler in the management of patients with subarachnoid haemorrhage: a review. *Acta Neurochir* 1999; **72** (Suppl.): 59–71.

25. Soustiel JF, Shik V, Shreiber R, *et al*. Basilar vasospasm diagnosis: investigation of a modified "Lindegaard Index" based on imaging studies and blood velocity measurements of the basilar artery. *Stroke* 2002; **33**: 72–7.

26. Sviri GE, Ghodke B, Britz GW, *et al*. Transcranial Doppler grading criteria for basilar artery vasospasm. *Neurosurgery* 2006; **59**: 360–6.

27. Aaslid R, Markwalder TM, Nornes H. Noninvasive transcranial Doppler ultrasound recording of flow velocity in basal cerebral arteries. *J Neurosurg* 1982; **57**: 769–74.

28. Lysakowski C, Walder B, Costanza MC, *et al*. Transcranial Doppler versus angiography in patients with vasospasm due to a ruptured cerebral aneurysm: A systematic review. *Stroke* 2001; **32**: 2292–8.

29. Qureshi AI, Sung GY, Razumovsky AY, *et al*. Early identification of patients at risk for symptomatic vasospasm after aneurismal subrachnoid hemorrhage. *Crit Care Med* 2000; **28**: 984–90.

30. Alexandrov AV, Sloan MA, Wong LKS, *et al*. Practice standards for transcranial Doppler (TCD) ultrasound. Part I. Test performance. *J Neuroimaging* 2007; **17**: 11–18.

31. Sloan MA. Transcranial Doppler monitoring of vasospasm after subarachnoid hemorrhage. In: Tegeler CH, Babikian VL, Gomez CR (eds). *Neurosonology*. St Louis: Mosby, 1996, pp. 156–71.

32. Sloan MA, Alexandrov AV, Tegeler CH, *et al*; Therapeutics and Technology Assessment Subcommittee of the American Academy of Neurology. Assessment: transcranial Doppler ultrasonography: report of the Therapeutics and Technology Assessment Subcommittee of

the American Academy of Neurology. *Neurology* 2004; **62**: 1468–81.

33. Spencer MP. Transcranial Doppler monitoring and causes of stroke from carotid endarterectomy. *Stroke* 1997; **28**: 685–91.

34. Rubiera M, Cava L, Tsivgoulis G, *et al*. Diagnostic criteria and yield of real time transcranial Doppler (TCD) monitoring of intra-arterial (IA) reperfusion procedures. *Stroke* 2010; **41**: 695–9.

35. Becker HM. Steal effect: natural principle of the collateralization of flow of arterial occlusions. *Med Klin* 1969; **64**: 882–6 [German].

36. Voigt K, Kendel K, Sauer M. Subclavian steal syndrome. Bloodless diagnosis of the syndrome using ultrasonic pulse echo and vertebral artery compression. *Fortschr Neurol Psychiatr Grenzgeb* 1970; **38**: 20–33 [German].

37. Alexandrov AV, Sharma VK, Lao AY, *et al*. Reversed Robin Hood syndrome in acute ischemic stroke patients. *Stroke* 2007; **38**: 3045–8.

10 Integration of Information and Case-Based Problem Solving

"Find reasons to treat."

A curative approach to stroke care

The initial evaluation of patients with acute cerebral ischemia is time sensitive, and the bedside examination should provide quick answers to the following key questions.

1. Is there a disabling deficit?
2. What is the mechanism of the event?
3. Can the damage be reversed?
4. Is the patient at risk of deterioration?

After ascertaining that the deficit is new and disabling, I consider treatment options to reverse the damage, and initiate treatment as soon as possible. I then set out to monitor the patient's condition and responses, if any, and prepare for the "worst case" scenario. Given the mechanism of any particular stroke, and if symptoms persist despite treatment, or if the patient's condition deteriorates, what would be my next step in treatment? What is the prognosis for the patient? I keep my multidisciplinary team as well as the patient or their family informed of my findings, what I am doing and why, and what to expect next. Though it sounds logical and simple, an emergency such as stroke leaves us little time, while our abilities to diagnose and monitor cerebral ischemia need further improvement.

Making a decision to start systemic tPA therapy, based on the disabling nature of the neurological deficit, CT scan showing no bleeding, and current time from symptom onset in relation to the treatment window, is the first step in learning stroke therapies. To me, stroke treatment duty does not end with delivery of tPA bolus. In fact, it is just the beginning.

Organizing care to deliver systemic tPA was the first curative task physicians faced in starting to care proactively (as opposed to reactively and only attending to complications, rehabilitation, and prevention needs) for stroke victims. Centers that managed to raise awareness and treat all eligible patients arriving on time are now looking to expand indications, explore combinatory treatments, and reach out to others – strides that will yield new approaches as long as we keep advancing our abilities to urgently evaluate and monitor this complex condition. Furthermore, stroke patients need to reach hospitals that provide care beyond just systemic tPA and conduct clinical trials and probe new approaches as a prerequisite to the development and implementation of newer therapies.

We have also made progress in understanding that transient ischemic attack (TIA) is an emergency [1, 2]. If a patient resolved the neurological symptoms spontaneously, this is encouraging indeed. However, a large proportion of patients with TIAs will proceed to have a stroke, and early preventative action is much needed [1–3]. In my response to a request for urgent evaluation, I do not ask the referring service such as Emergency Medicine to differentiate TIA versus persisting symptoms. Half jokingly, I say that I run even faster if symptoms resolve or are improving acutely because this demonstrates that the patient has "recoverable" brain tissues.

If a deficit persists or recurs, our system is geared up for a fast and standardized evaluation to determine candidacy for treatment. It should be "well oiled" and performing consistently, day and night. This chapter will describe information obtainable by clinical observation and ultrasound at the bedside in addition to the NIHSS score and complimentary to multimodal CT or MRI. This additional information can be integrated with the rest of the protocols, and sometimes could provide that pivotal "a-ha!" moment.

Neurovascular Examination: The Rapid Evaluation of Stroke Patients Using Ultrasound Waveform Interpretation, First Edition.
Andrei V. Alexandrov.
© 2013 Andrei V. Alexandrov. Published 2013 by Blackwell Publishing Ltd.

Case study 10.1 Early neurological deterioration

A 55-year-old over-weight woman with a history of untreated obstructive sleep apnea (OSA) and arterial hypertension presented with fluctuating left-sided weakness that started earlier that day [4]. On admission, she had mild left-sided hemiparesis and facial palsy with dysarthria (NIHSS score = 6). Non-contrast CT showed hyperdense MCA sign (Figure 10.1). TCD showed a blunted residual flow signal (TIBI 2) in the right proximal M1 MCA (Figure 10.1) indicating an MCA occlusion. Intravenous tPA was started 200 minutes after the initial symptom onset and TCD showed velocity improvement and partial recanalization towards the end of tPA infusion (Figure 10.1).

At the end of tPA infusion, the patient developed excessive sleepiness with repetitive episodes (each lasting approximately 30 seconds) of irregular breathing and desaturation (with oxygen saturation levels below 90% under 2 to 4 liters supplemental oxygen delivered by a nasal cannula). Her neuro-

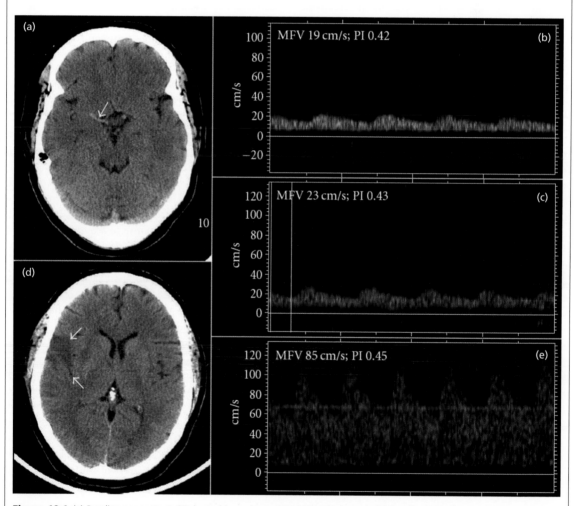

Figure 10.1 (**a**) Baseline noncontrast CT showed hyperdense right M1 MCA (arrow). (**b**) Baseline TCD: flattened systolic flow acceleration (TIBI 2) at a depth of 48 mm, indicating right proximal MCA occlusion. (**c**) Improved flow velocities indicate a slow and partial recanalization just before clinical deterioration. (**d**) Follow-up CT showed a cortical infarction (arrows). (**e**) A 24-hour TCD: normal flow velocities and waveforms (TIBI 5) at a depth of 46 mm indicating complete recanalization.

logical symptoms worsened rapidly in less than 1 minute to complete left-sided plegia and a total NIHSS score of 24 points. Her blood pressure and heart rate ranged from 126/61 mmHg to 164/93 mmHg and 72 to 98 bpm, respectively, during the entire monitoring period, and did not drop significantly during the neurological worsening.

An urgent CT (completed within 15 minutes after neurological worsening) ruled out intracerebral hemorrhage and edema progression. TCD monitoring showed persisting right MCA occlusion (TIBI score 2) and paradoxical as well as transient velocity decreases (by >10 cm/s) during hypoventilation episodes, consistent with intracranial blood flow steal (as described in previous chapters).

Because of the continuation of excessive sleepiness with apnea periods, the patient was placed on bilevel positive airway pressure (BPAP). Within the next hour, the patient improved to an NIHSS score of 13.

At 24 hours, CT demonstrated a cortical infarct in the right MCA territory (Figure 10.1). On TCD, the right MCA appeared completely recanalized (TIBI score 5, Figure 10.1). Further clinical workup revealed a moderate 50–69% stenosis of the right internal carotid artery strongly suggesting large-artery thrombosis and artery-to-artery embolism as the likely mechanism of her stroke. BPAP was transitioned to night-time ventilation only, and her neurological status improved to an NIHSS of 6 at discharge.

One month later, she had a residual minor left-sided hemiparesis and was functionally independent (NIHSS 3, modified Rankin Scale 1). An overnight sleep study demonstrated a significant obstructive sleep apnea (OSA, apnea–hypopnea index >10/h) for which she started on portable noninvasive ventilatory correction at home.

Comment: Problem solving in this case stretched beyond the standard of care that would have required only repeat CT, flat head-of-bed positioning, hydration, and allowing BP to be up to (but not exceeding) 180/100 mmHg post-tPA. An alternative option to that carried out here would have been to consider bridging i.v. tPA with an intra-arterial (IA) procedure for persisting arterial occlusion, given its hemodynamic significance and severe neurological worsening. This could have been an option if we had firm proof that this approach is superior to just i.v. tPA alone or if this patient was not already enrolled into another hyperacute trial of the pharmacological augmentation of systemic tPA action precluding IA procedures. Ultrasound demonstration of the hemodynamic significance of hypoventilation episodes helped choose early initiation of noninvasive ventilatory correction that, presumably, through removal of carbon dioxide secured some collaterals and maintained the residual flow leading to some neurological improvement despite persistence of the arterial occlusion.

Case study 10.2 Lack of recovery despite proximal recanalization

A 43-year-old woman presented with "altered mental status" to an outside hospital where she was initially treated for a suspected partial complex seizure and transferred to our center once stroke was suspected. Upon arrival, she is arousable, does not speak, follows occasional commands, right extremities 2/5, left extremities 4/5 strength, and she has gaze preference to the left that she was able to overcome. Total NIHSS score = 17. Noncontrast CT was normal at the outside hospital, however the patient did not receive systemic tPA due to concerns for a seizure and subsequently for the time elapsed from symptom onset.

On TCD, both the right and left MCAs had normal (TIBI 5) flows in the M1 segments. The neurological status, however, was not improving. Also during TCD examination, clusters of microembolic signals were noticed (Figure 10.2). The clusters contained on average 10–20 signals and reoccurred spontaneously every 20–30 seconds. These TCD findings were

(Continued)

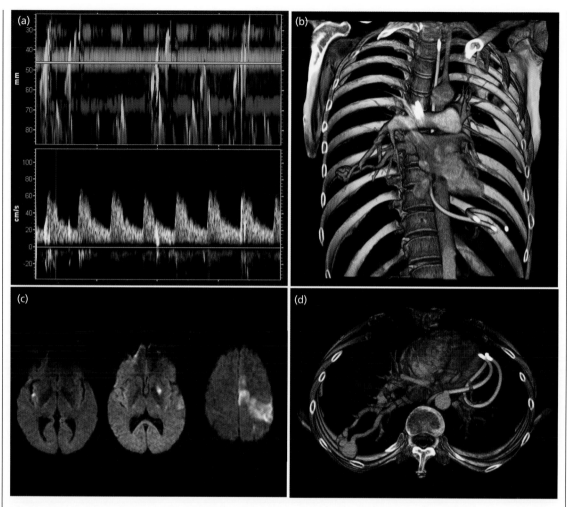

Figure 10.2 (**a**) PMD TCD findings of spontaneous embolic signals with relatively wide signatures on M-mode suggesting longer transit times at any given depth/gate, a sign of large-size air bubbles in the setting of a right-to-left shunt at rest. (**b**) Reconstructed CTA of the chest show a large pulmonary AVM. (**c, d**) Bihemispheric embolic strokes on DWI.

consistent with the right-to-left shunt present at rest. Given the number of intravenous injections, medicine administrations, saline volume, and overall infusions that patient has received, gaseous brain embolism was suspected in addition to an ischemic embolic event likely in the presence of a right-to-left shunt.

The patient was urgently sent to a hyperbaric chamber for treatment of cerebral air embolism. After a 2-hour long treatment (pressure at depth 60 feet of sea water), no recurrent embolic signals were detectable on TCD, and the patient became alert and started to follow commands consistently. DWI showed the extent of her lesions in both left and right hemispheres (Figure 10.2). Echocardiography did not show an intracardiac shunt while CT-angiography of the chest showed a large pulmonary arteriovenous malformation (PAVM) (Figure 10.2). PAVM was subsequently closed percutaneously. Hypercoagulable and genetic work-ups were negative. Her NIHSS at discharge to rehabilitation was 8 (expressive aphasia and moderate weakness). Her NIHSS at 3 months was 2 (mild word finding difficulties) and mRS of 1.

Comment: Poor arousability, inability to speak, and overall neurological findings that did not fit just one arterial territory can arise from the posterior circulation lesions or can be due to bihemispheric embolization. However, the patient was disproportionately disabled given the size and location of lesions on DWI. The usual suspects could be seizures, systemic hypotension, or hypoxemia with a significant shunt. While she received antiepileptic medicines at an outside hospital with no neurological improvement, her BP remained stable and her oxygen saturation was normal during the acute phase. Emboli causing her strokes went into distal vasculature and the proximal vessels were patent, precluding the need for IA procedures at an extended time window. Thus, TCD findings of multiple air microbubbles entering the brain circulation repeatedly was concerning and helpful in deciding on further management steps as it gave us a potential therapeutic target – ongoing cerebral air embolism. The reason for this is the size of air bubbles introduced with intravenous infusions. During echocardiography or the so-called TCD "bubble" test for a right-to-left shunt, we create air bubbles that are about 40–60 micron in size by agitating 9 cc normal saline with 1 cc air between two syringes via a three-way stop-cock connector [5]. In this more-or-less controlled environment air bubbles are microscopically small, yet they are larger than lung capillaries (usually 8–12 microns in diameter). When these air bubbles are not cleared by the lungs and sneak through a shunt, we detect them by ultrasound as either paradoxically appearing in the left heart chambers on echo, or in the MCA with TCD [6]. Once we see those signals present at rest during TCD in an acute stroke patient, the patient either has an artificial valve, or a thromboemboligenic surface such as an ulcerated plaque or intraluminal proximal thrombus, or gaseous brain embolization. Thus, routine infusion of saline or medicines with repeated flushes during acute management of our patient could have created large air bubbles that would pass unobstructed through our patient's PAVM (see the size of the feeding and draining vessels on CTA in Figure 10.2).

Even though hyperbaric oxygenation has not been adequately tested in the acute phase of cerebral ischemia, our choice of this treatment was guided by the real-time proof of air embolization that was ongoing, not by persistence of symptoms despite patent proximal vessels. Whether this procedure could have contributed to fostering early neurological recovery will remain unknown (until we are able to properly test this or comparable treatments in acute stroke); however, the early progress she made directly after the procedure was encouraging to see.

Case study 10.3 Stroke in a patient with known hypercoagulable disorder

A 24-year-old man had a history of recurrent deep venous thrombosis and was taken off warfarin for a dental procedure. No anticoagulation was initiated postprocedure and the patient was not instructed to restart taking warfarin. He presented with a progressive 4-day history of weakness in his left distal arm. Admission head CT scan is positive for a small cortical hypoattenuation and no systemic tPA was given. His NIHSS score was 4 (accounting for 1/5 distal arm and mild sensory loss; no cortical signs).

Carotid duplex in the emergency room demonstrated a lesion in the right ICA bulb that produces a severe stenosis (Figure 10.3). It appeared to be a partially recanalized thrombus with no pre-existing plaque formation. MRI DWI was completed next to visualize the extent of his stroke (Figure 10.4). Upon discussion of risks, the patient and family agreed to restart anticoagulation with enoxaparin and warfarin. The patient was monitored with neurological examinations every 2 hours and TCD emboli detection once daily while receiving acute rehabilitation in our hospital. His NIHSS decreased to 1 on day 4, and he was sent home on enoxaparin/ warfarin. INR reached therapeutic levels in 11 days, enoxaparin was stopped, and he continues taking warfarin. His repeat carotid duplex ultrasound showed complete thrombus resolution at 1.5 months after stroke.

(Continued)

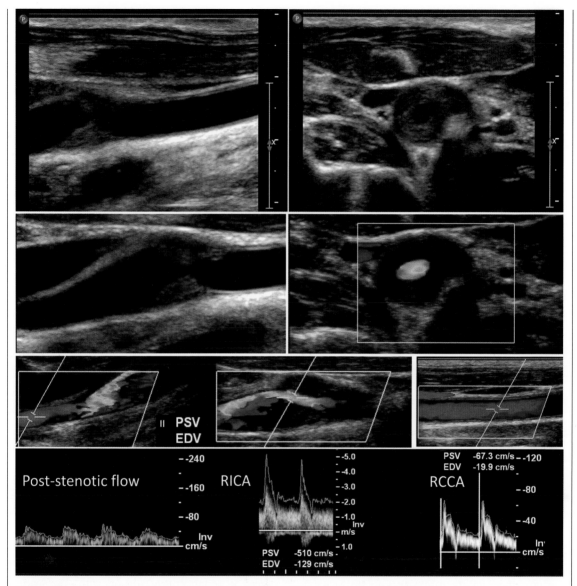

Figure 10.3 Longitudinal and transverse B-mode images of a soft thrombus in the carotid bulb without evidence of a pre-existing atheromatous disease with corresponding color flow images and spectral Doppler findings.

Comment: Knowing the location of an arterial lesion helps to ascertain a mismatch between what is already likely lost compared to what could be lost if reocclusion or thrombus propagation occur. With a minor deficit and propensity to form clots, one might suspect cortical arterial thrombosis that was extending over days producing a small stroke. The surprise was a thrombus (likely embolus) in the proximal ICA that partially recanalized on its own and was perhaps responsible for an artery-to-artery embolization or hemodynamic worsening overtime, producing the moderate size cortical lesion. Of note, MRI DWI and FLAIR sequences showed strokes of different age within this lesion (images not shown) with their localization favoring both mechanisms, embolic and hemodynamic, that continued after the initial thrombus lodging into the right ICA bulb. Even though these comments remain speculative,

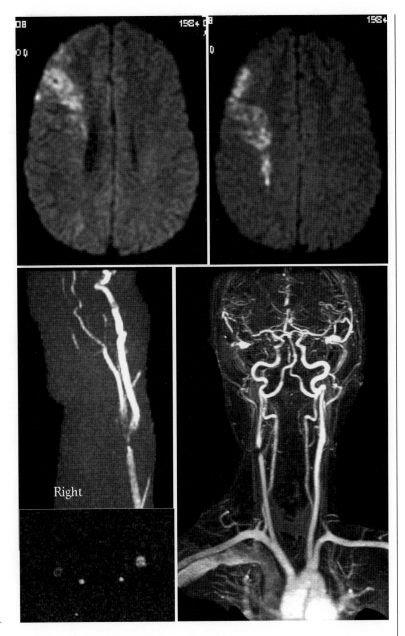

Figure 10.4 DWI and MRA findings.

the knowledge of a large thrombus presence, the severe stenosis across it, and a larger brain territory at potential risk was helpful to explain why and how stroke developed in this young person, and why risks of restarting anticoagulation by bridging appear justified. Ultrasound also provided a noninvasive surveillance tool to see if thrombus dissolution would take a more aggressive turn (emboli detection). Together with neurological examinations, it offered a noninvasive way of monitoring thrombus dissolution and any re-occlusion or embolization requiring an intervention (i.e. surgical thrombectomy or catheter intra-arterial rescue at an extended time window).

Case study 10.4 Neurological worsening after delayed proximal recanalization

A 73-year-old man with a history of arterial hyper- tension and smoking arrived to our Emergency Department at 1 hour from sudden onset of left- sided weakness. His noncontrast CT scan showed no hypoattenuation, no hemorrhage, and age-expected atrophy (Figure 10.5). His NIHSS score was 12. He received intravenous tPA and recovered to a total NIHSS score of 3 points by the end of tPA infusion. He remained stable with mild inattention to the left side and arm drift (NIHSS 3) for 2 days while in hos- pital. His vascular imaging during this time showed a complete proximal ICA occlusion with a fresh throm- bus, irregular heart rhythm due to atrial fibrillation (Figure 10.6), and a cortical embolic stroke in the posterior right MCA subdivision (Figure 10.5). At 48 hours, neurological worsening was found during stroke team rounds. He was looking away from his left side and his left arm was plegic. He followed com- mands with his left leg, which had a strength of 4/5 (total NIHSS score was 9, also due to redevelopment of dysarthria and left-sided facial weakness). Carotid ultrasound at the bedside showed partial recanaliza- tion of his right ICA thrombus on the neck (Figure 10.7) while TCD shows a tandem lesion in the right M1 MCA (TIBI 2 blunted signal, MFV <20 cm/s, image not shown). Urgent head CT/CT-perfusion showed no bleeding, the presence of hypoattenua- tion corresponding to his prior acute stroke present

on DWI, and a large area of hypoperfusion involving the entire right MCA territory (Figure 10.8). Catheter angiogram confirmed ultrasound findings and the decision was made to surgically excise the right ICA thrombus first (Figure 10.9). After thrombectomy, no embolus is seen in the M1 segment and anterior M2 subdivision of the right MCA on catheter angiogra- phy (images not shown). His NIHSS improved to 4 points and he was discharged to rehabilitation 7 days after the initial stroke.

Comment: delayed and partial recanalization of a proximal thrombus can cause distal embolization and neurological worsening. Its occurrence without full prior recovery or within 3 months after the index stroke currently precludes administration of systemic tPA [7]. The questions were: (a) where is the offending lesion, and (b) does a proximal throm- bus still exist or did it completely move intracrani- ally? A quick bedside carotid duplex scan provided the shortest path to these answers. The next ques- tion was: is there brain tissue at risk outside the area already affected by the subacute stroke? The neuro- logical examination, showing a new and disabling deficit, as well as noncontrast CT scan, showing hypoattenuation not extending beyond what was seen on DWI, made such a conclusion likely. CT- perfusion was done to visualize the new perfusion

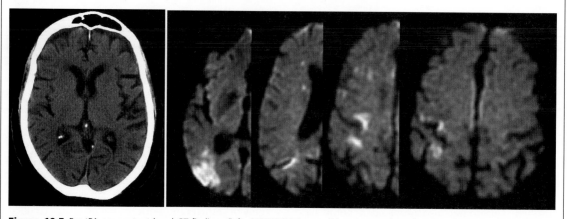

Figure 10.5 Pre-tPA noncontrast head CT findings (left, ASPECTS 10, rest of images not shown) and post tPA DWI findings of an embolic infarct in the posterior right MCA subdivision.

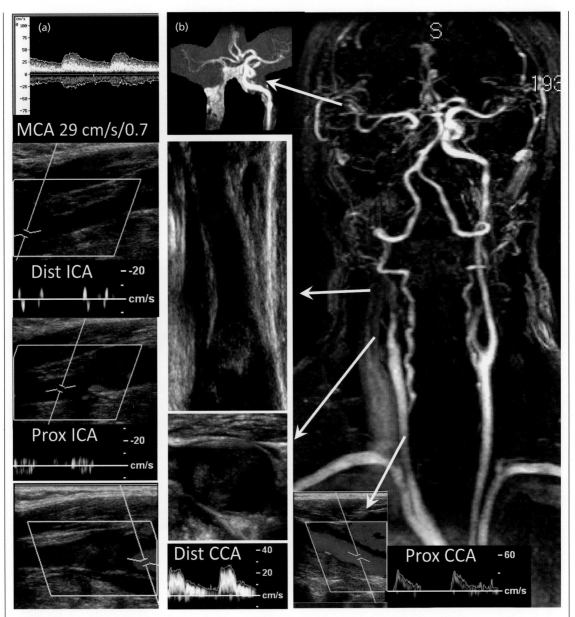

Figure 10.6 (a) Top image shows blunted right MCA waveform in the setting of a proximal hemodynamically significant ICA obstruction. (a) Images demonstrate the carotid duplex showing a complete ICA occlusion with a fresh thrombus. (b) Corresponding MRA findings.

(Continued)

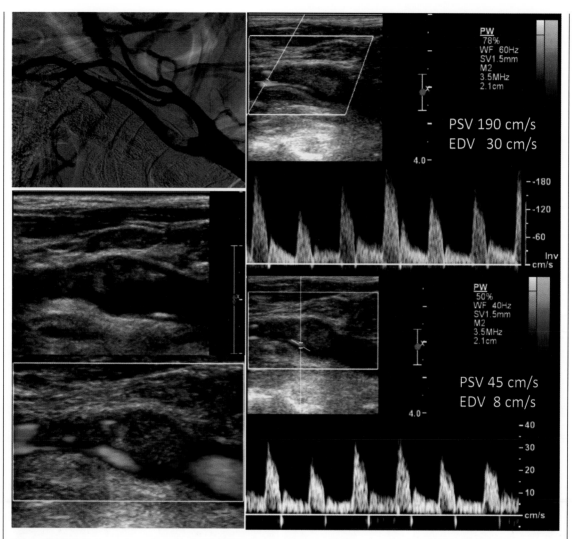

Figure 10.7 Catheter angiography and carotid duplex ultrasound images showing recanalization of the ICA thrombus.

deficit and all imaging information was used to explain why the new stroke happened, what can be done at this extended time window, and to obtain consent for carotid thrombectomy for an acute ischemic deficit. Although several case reports indicated the risk of complication of this operation, a recent single-center experience suggested that both urgent CEA and carotid thrombectomy can be done with acceptable safety [8]. As fortunately happened in this case, surgical thrombectomy of the proximal ICA lesion improved blood flow to the brain and helped to spontaneously lyse the intracranial tandem lesion, thus eliminating the need for further risky interventions.

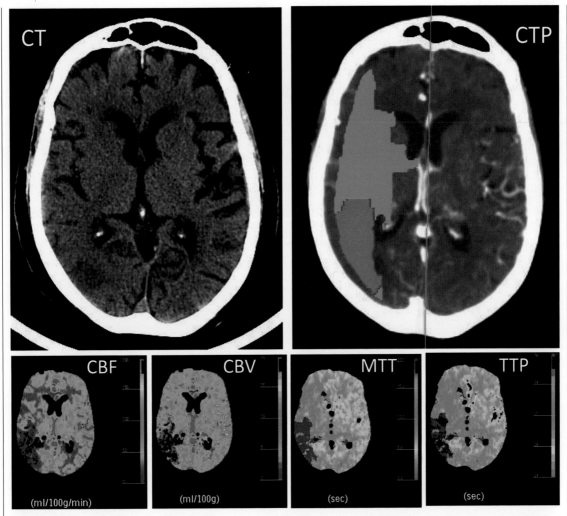

Figure 10.8 CT-perfusion findings and prognostic maps (red indicates likely irreversibly damaged and green indicates potentially salvageable brain tissues) CBF, cerebral blood flow; CBV, cerebral blood flow volume; MTT, mean transit time; TTP, time to peak.

(Continued)

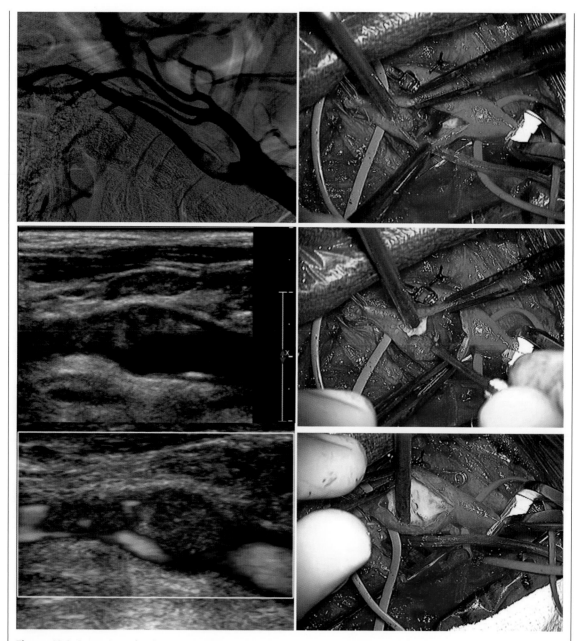

Figure 10.9 Comparison of catheter angiography, carotid duplex, and intraoperative findings during ICA thrombectomy.

Case study 10.5 A lesion in the distal common carotid artery

A 75-year-old woman with a history of arterial hypertension, atrial fibrillation (not on an antico-agulant), and functionally independent prior to her current stroke, received intravenous tPA for a new-onset left-sided weakness (total NIHSS 12 points) with no early recovery. She underwent MRI/MRA (Figure 10.10) that showed a large ischemic stroke in the right MCA and a right common carotid artery occlusion with reconstituted flow in the right ICA distally. She proceeded with inpatient rehabilitation and recovered the left leg function more than the arm to a total NIHSS score of 7 points. Ultrasound findings showed the following (Figure 10.10):

1. a soft and long thrombus extending from the proximal CCA;
2. mixed long atherosclerotic plaque in the distal CCA and its bifurcation;
3. complete CCA occlusion;
4. reversed ECA flow (images not shown);
5. antegrade ICA flow with tardus parvus (blunted signal).

Catheter angiography confirmed ultrasound findings and carotid endarterectomy with thrombectomy was performed 4 weeks after her stroke. The patient remained neurologically unchanged and was transferred to an inpatient rehabilitation facility.

Comment: an occlusion in the common carotid artery may not necessarily obstruct the ICA flow, and interrogation of a vessel distal to the occlusion site should be performed when feasible [9]. The ICA flow could be reversed to supply the ECA, and vice versa if the circle of Willis is incompetent. The presence of an ICA flow makes the occlusion segmental, excisable, or suitable for a bypass surgery [10]. The contributions of ultrasound in this case were to demonstrate that fresh thrombus in the CCA was not the only lesion, and the overall extent of the diseased segment of vasculature on the neck. There was also a pre-existing atheroma in the distal portion making the stroke mechanism either large-vessel atherothrombotic or cardioembolic with an embolus that lodged in the distal CCA. In both scenarios (*in situ* thrombosis with proximal propagation or an embolus), pre-existing stenosis in the distal CCA likely played a protective role as it allowed ECA flow to reverse and maintain flow into the ICA. Her wedge-shape MCA stroke was therefore most likely an artery-to-artery embolism with a fragment of the thrombus or an embolus.

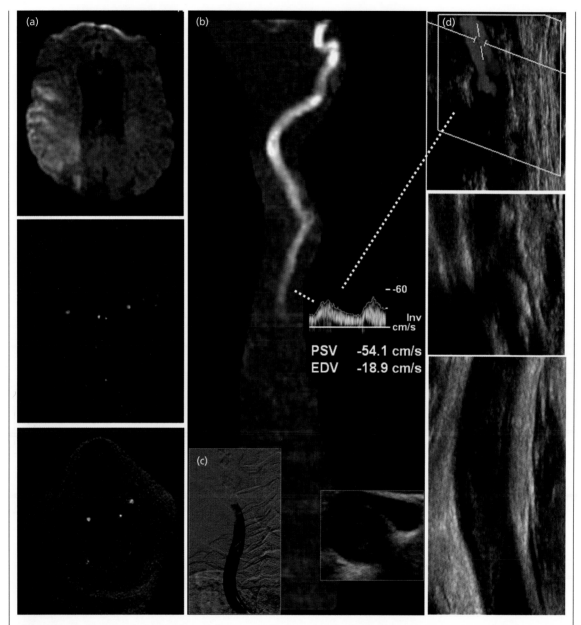

Figure 10.10 DWI, MRA findings (**a**, **b**), catheter angiography (**c**), and corresponding carotid duplex ultrasound findings (**d**) showing CCA occlusion with a large thrombus, pre-existing distal CCA atheroma, and complete occlusion with reconstituted ICA flow distal to CCA obstruction.

Case study 10.6 Unstable intracranial stenosis

A 54-year-old African-American woman with a history of arterial hypertension, breast cancer, and transient ischemic attack presented to our Emergency Department with new-onset loss of vision, left-sided headache, nausea, emesis, and disorientation, which started 2 days ago [11]. Her admission neurological examination showed residual light perception, bilateral horizontal nystagmus, and no motor weakness (NIHSS score 4). PMD-TCD showed a blunted flow signal (TIBI grade 2) in the proximal

BA compatible with a flow-limiting BA stenosis (Figure 10.11). MRA also showed a significant stenosis in the proximal BA (images not shown). MRI showed bilateral infarctions in occipital lobes and cerebellum (Figure 10.11). The patient received aspirin 325 mg and clopidogrel 300 mg load followed by aspirin 325 mg and clopidogrel 75 mg daily. Her symptoms improved over 3 days with return of object recognition while vision field loss became limited to a right-sided homonymous hemianopsia (NIHSS 2).

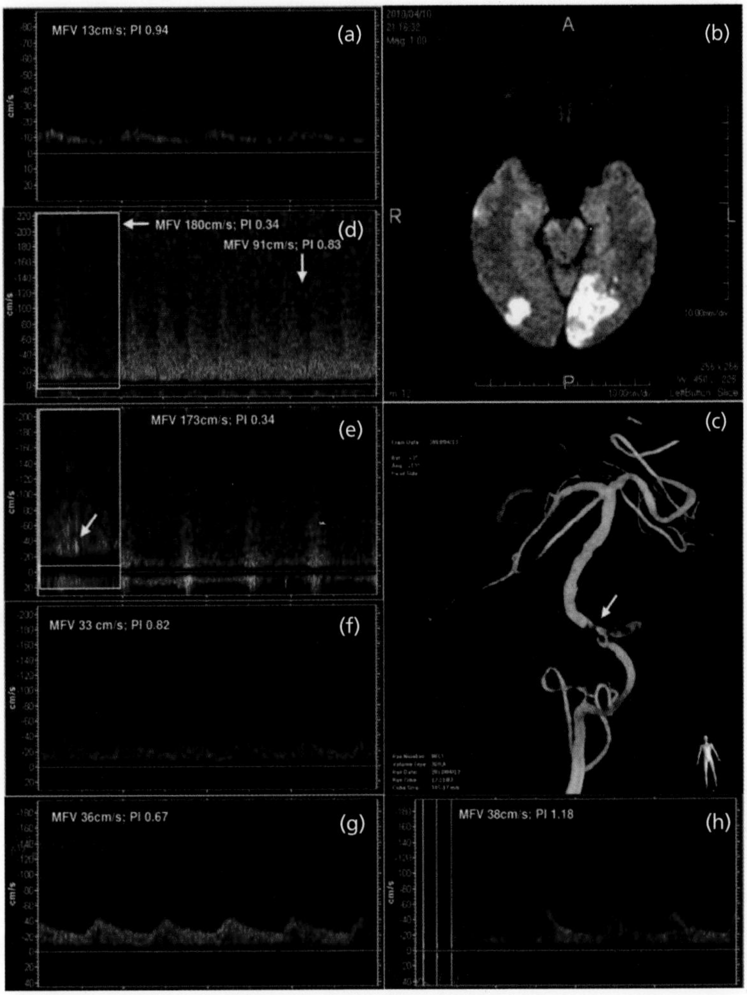

Figure 10.11 (a) Baseline TCD: delayed systolic flow acceleration (TIBI 2) at a depth of 81 mm, indicating high-grade proximal BA stenosis. (b) MRI: diffusion restriction in both PCAs (left > right). (c) Catheter angiography: three-dimensional reconstruction of a severe irregular-surface proximal BA stenosis (arrow). (d) TCD: improved mean flow velocity in the proximal BA at 80 mm (insert left) and possible hyperemic reperfusion of the distal BA at 99 mm. (e) High-velocity turbulent flow and microemboli (insert left) in the mid-BA at 92 mm. (f) Decreased flow velocity with delayed systolic flow acceleration in the mid-BA at 87 mm. (g, h) Blunted flow signals at the proximal and mid-BA segments 24 hours after administration of dextran-40.

(Continued)

Catheter angiography 3 days after admission showed a severe and irregular-surface proximal BA stenosis originating from the terminal right vertebral artery (Figure 10.11). One hour after catheter angiography, the patient complained of severe (10/10) headache, her systolic blood pressure was 240 mmHg. However, she had no new focal deficits. At this point, PMD-TCD showed improved mean flow velocity (TIBI grade 4 flow, MFV 180 cm/s) in the proximal BA, indicating recanalization and possible hyperemic reperfusion of the distal vasculature (distal BA, MFV 91 cm/s; Figure 10.11). Headache resolved with systolic blood pressure lowering to 175 mmHg with nicardipine.

One hour later, the patient developed vertigo and left-sided ataxia. She started to fluctuate with NIHSS changing from 2 to 6 points followed by an episode of unresponsiveness. Her blood pressure was 170 mmHg. Urgent noncontrast CT showed no intracerebral hemorrhage (images not shown). PMD-TCD showed embolic signals in the proximal BA along with a high-velocity jet in the middle BA (TIBI grade 4 flow, MFV 173 cm/s), suggestive of artery-to-artery embolization and thrombus movement along the BA stem (Figure 10.11). We initiated intravenous dextran-40 infusion (20 mL/h over 24 hours). During the next hour, flow velocities through the proximal and mid-BA decreased to 33–46 cm/s with delayed systolic flow acceleration and no microembolic signals (Figure 10.11). The patient's symptoms resolved back to the NIHSS score of 2 with no subsequent fluctuation. At 24 hours, PMD-TCD showed low-velocity/ delayed systolic flow acceleration signals throughout its entire stem (MFV 36–39 cm/s, Figure 10.11), while MRI/MRA showed persistence of the proximal BA stenosis and no new parenchymal lesions. The patient experienced no side effects during or after the dextran-40 infusion. At the time of discharge, the patient's only deficit was a right-sided homonymous hemianopsia. Two months later, at an outpatient visit, she had no neurological deficit and was functionally independent without any assistance (NIHSS 0, modified Rankin Scale 0).

Comment: This case highlights a dilemma about how to manage patients with persisting arterial stenoses, artery-to-artery embolization, and re-occlusion, particularly in the setting of evolving or subacute infarction. The Stenting versus Aggressive Medical Management for Stroke Prevention in Patients with Intracranial Arterial Stenosis (SAMMPRIS) trial showed no advantage of intracranial stenting over best medical therapy [12] but these findings apply to patients after stroke or TIA who were stable for 72 hours or more. Of note, this patient experienced these events while already receiving dual antiplatelet therapy and statin. A further problem was related to how to manage her blood pressure. Severe headache (and likely underlying hyperperfusion mechanism with excessively high blood pressure) required blood pressure lowering while persisting high-grade BA stenosis and thrombus moving through the BA stem prompted us not to lower it too low. TCD provided real-time insight into the pathogenesis of her symptoms and potential ways to stabilize the situation. Hypothetically, to achieve a compromise between lower blood pressure and maintenance of brain perfusion, volume expansion could be an option. The high molecular weight polysaccharide dextran-40 provides volume expansion and it also has mild antithrombotic properties [13, 14]. It has been safely applied in patients with extracranial atherosclerotic disease undergoing CEA, effectively reducing postoperative Doppler-detectable microembolization due to its antithrombotic and antiplatelet effect [13–15]. With new real-time monitoring tools at hand, the issue of volume expanders in acute phase of ischemia could perhaps be revisited.

Case study 10.7 Whole body shaking TIAs

A 49-year-old right-handed White man with a history of smoking, arterial hypertension, and obstructive sleep apnea has had numerous seizure-like episodes of whole body shaking (without facial involvement) that interfered with his ability to work over the past 5 years [16]. These episodes had increased in frequency and severity over recent months while lasting for few seconds up to 1 minute. Prolonged standing, raising hands, climbing stairs, and walking precipitated these attacks. Body shaking stopped after falling or lying down. Consciousness was not impaired during the attacks. One day prior to admission, he developed left facial droop, dysarthria, and left arm weakness. His NIHSS score upon arrival was 4 points. Cerebral computed tomography (CT) showed cortical hypodensity in the right frontal lobe. Episodes of whole body shaking continued in the hospital. His blood pressure and heart rate remained stable and did not drop significantly during episodes of whole body shaking. Long-term video electroencephalography during the attacks showed mild-to-moderate diffuse slowing, but no epileptiform transients and no electrographic seizure. His MRI showed bilateral frontoparietal and cortical watershed infarcts of different age and occlusions in the left common carotid artery, bilateral internal carotid arteries, as well as a severe left vertebral artery (VA) origin stenosis (Figure 10.12). Catheter angiogram showed that the right VA was the only contributor to collateralization of flow from the posterior to anterior circulation via posterior communicating arteries as well as leptomeningeal vessels and posterior pericallosal artery producing reversed flow in both anterior cerebral arteries (Figure 10.12). TCD showed blunted waveforms in both MCAs with velocities paradoxically decreasing bilaterally indicating hypercapnia-induced blood flow steal in response to voluntary breath holding (Figure 10.12). The magnitude of steal for the right and left MCA was −35.5% and −25.6%, respectively, leading to a neurological deterioration with a 2 point increment increase in the NIHSS score for the leg and arm motor strength during steal episodes.

Angioplasty of the severe stenosis of the left VA origin was performed on day one of the hospital stay in an attempt to restore its capacity to contribute to the collateral flow supply. He also received atorvastatin 80 mg daily, combined antiplatelet therapy (aspirin and clopidogrel) for 1 month, followed by clopidogrel monotherapy as well as smoking cessation counseling. From admission, the patient was placed on continuous positive airway pressure (CPAP) ventilatory assistance for 3 days in the hospital. In the following days, neurological fluctuation no longer occurred. The patient was instructed to use CPAP at night for his sleep apnea after a formal sleep study was conducted postdischarge.

After 6 months, he returned for follow up and reported no further episodes of body shaking. His NIHSS score was 1 (mild arm weakness) and his mRS score was 0. He stated that he exercises daily with brisk walking up to 2 miles. On repeat TCD, vasomotor reactivity remained significantly impaired; however, MCA velocities started to increase in response to breath holding (breath-holding index: right MCA = 0, left MCA = 0.31) with no steal effect seen (Figure 10.12).

Comment: this case helped us to describe a whole body shaking syndrome [16] which appears to be a bilateral form of the one-sided limb shaking phenomena seen with hypoperfusion distal to the contralateral carotid artery occlusion [17–20]. The three-vessel occlusion and the severe stenosis in the forth major precerebral vessel made both of our patient's motor strips become vulnerable to episodes of hypoperfusion and steal. Multimodal evaluation of this patient showed that despite recruitment of collateral channels, his collateral supply was fragile while his risk factors remained uncontrolled. As currently thought best, medical therapy was

(Continued)

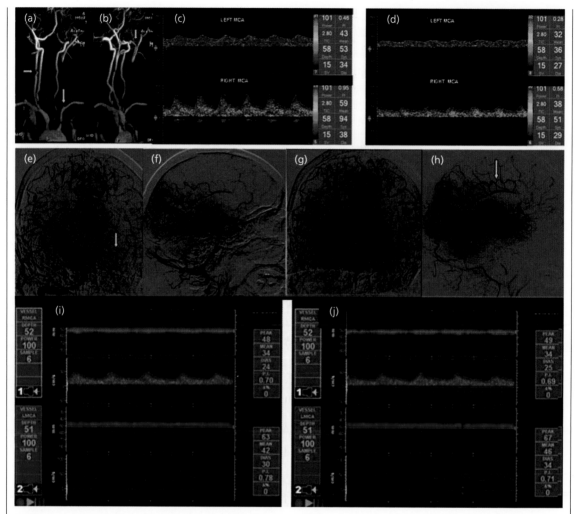

Figure 10.12 (**a**, **b**) MRA shows occlusions: right ICA, left ICA, left CCA, and left origin VA stenosis (arrows). Left external carotid artery-to-VA anastomosis (arrow on panel b). (**c**, **d**) TCD during normocapnia (**c**) and hypercapnia (**d**) showing bilateral steal. (**e–h**) Right vertebral injection showing posterior communicating artery, collateral flow, and reversed ACA (arrows). (**i**, **j**) Breath holding test after 6 months (right MCA no change; left MCA velocity improvement with hypercapnia).

instituted and an experimental dilation of the severely stenosed vertebral artery (that could potentially be an additional contributor to the collateral supply) was performed but the vessel was found to have become restenosed 24 hours later on repeat ultrasound examination (data not shown, no stent was placed). Noninvasive ventilatory correction appeared pivotal as neurological fluctuations stopped during the next several days while the key to long-term success was likely physical exercise and risk factor control, in addition to medical therapy.

Conclusion

We continue our journey to better understand how stroke occurs, how the brain becomes damaged, and how it manages to survive or triumph if the right aid is delivered on time. In my opinion, real-time physiological assessment together with structural imaging is the way to move forward, with the aim of tailoring treatment to individual patient conditions. The treatment of stroke provides a vast opportunity for clinicians and scientists to explore options for these procedures.

References

1. Johnston SC, Gress DR, Browner WS, et al. Short-term prognosis after emergency department diagnosis of TIA. JAMA 2000; 284: 2901–6.

2. Johnston SC, Rothwell PM, Nguyen-Huynh MN, et al. Validation and refinement of scores to predict very early stroke risk after transient ischaemic attack. Lancet 2007; 369: 283–92.

3. Rothwell PM, Giles MF, Chandratheva A, et al. Early use of Existing Preventive Strategies for Stroke (EXPRESS) study. Effect of urgent treatment of transient ischaemic attack and minor stroke on early recurrent stroke (EXPRESS study): a prospective population-based sequential comparison. Lancet 2007; 370: 1432–42.

4. Barlinn K, Balucani C, Palazzo P, et al. Noninvasive ventilatory correction as an adjunct to an experimental systemic reperfusion therapy in acute ischemic stroke. Stroke Res Treat 2010: 108253.

5. Sharma VK, Tsivgoulis G, Lao AY, et al. Quantification of microspheres (μS) appearance in brain vessels: implications for residual flow velocity measurements, dose calculations and potential drug delivery. Stroke 2008; 39: 1476–81.

6. Jauss M, Zanette E. Detection of right-to-left shunt with ultrasound contrast agent and transcranial Doppler sonography. Cerebrovasc Dis 2003; 10: 490–6.

7. Adams HP Jr, del Zoppo G, Alberts MJ, et al. American Heart Association/American Stroke Association Stroke Council; American Heart Association/American Stroke Association Clinical Cardiology Council; American Heart Association/American Stroke Association Cardiovascular Radiology and Intervention Council; Atherosclerotic Peripheral Vascular Disease Working Group; Quality of Care Outcomes in Research Interdisciplinary Working Group. Guidelines for the early management of adults with ischemic stroke: a guideline from the American Heart Association/American Stroke Association Stroke Council, Clinical Cardiology Council, Cardiovascular Radiology and Intervention Council, and the Atherosclerotic Peripheral Vascular Disease and Quality of Care Outcomes in Research Interdisciplinary Working Groups: The American Academy of Neurology affirms the value of this guideline as an educational tool for neurologists. Circulation 2007; 115: e478–534.

8. Mussa FF, Aaronson N, Lamparello PJ, et al. Outcome of carotid endarterectomy for acute neurological deficit. Vasc Endovascular Surg 2009; 43: 364–9.

9. Bowen JC, Garcia M, Garrard CL, et al. Anomalous branch of the internal carotid artery maintains patency distal to a complete occlusion diagnosed by duplex scan. J Vasc Surg 1997; 26: 164–7.

10. Salam TA, Smith RB 3rd, Lumsden AB. Extrathoracic bypass procedures for proximal common carotid artery lesions. Am J Surg 1993; 166: 163–6.

11. Palazzo P, Barlinn K, Balucani C, et al. Potential role of PMD-TCD monitoring in the management of hemodynamically unstable intracranial stenosis. J Neuroimaging 2012; 22: 305–7.

12. Chimowitz MI, Lynn MJ, Derdeyn CP, et al. the SAMMPRIS Trial Investigators. Stenting versus aggressive medical therapy for intracranial arterial stenosis. N Engl J Med 2011; 365: 993–1003.

13. Abir F, Barkhordarian S, Sumpio BE. Efficacy of dextran solutions in vascular surgery. Vasc Endovascular Surg 2004; 38: 483–91.

14. Jones CI, Payne DA, Hayes PD, et al. The antithrombotic effect of dextran-40 in man is due to enhanced fibrinolysis in vivo. J Vasc Surg 2008; 48: 715–22.

15. Lennard NS, Vijayasekar C, Tiivas C, et al. Control of emboli in patients with recurrent or crescendo transient ischaemic attacks using preoperative transcranial Doppler-directed Dextran therapy. Br J Surg 2003; 90: 166–70.

16. Nguyen HT, Zhao L, Barlinn K, et al. Whole body shaking due to intracranial blood flow steal. J Neurol Sci 2011; 305: 165–6.

17. Fisher CM. Concerning recurrent transient cerebral ischemic attacks. Can Med Assoc J 1962; 86: 1091–9.

18. Persoon S, Kappelle LJ, Klijn CJ. Limb-shaking transient ischaemic attacks in patients with internal carotid artery occlusion: a case-control study. Brain 2010; 133: 915–22.

19. Baquis GD, Pessin MS, Scott RM. Limb shaking: a carotid TIA. Stroke 1985; 16: 444–8.

20. Tatemichi TK, Young WL, Prohovnik I, et al. Perfusion insufficiency in limb-shaking transient ischemic attack. Stroke 1990; 21: 341–7.

Index

Neurovascular Examination: The Rapid Evaluation of Stroke Patients Using Ultrasound Waveform Interpretation, First Edition. Andrei V. Alexandrov.
© 2013 Andrei V. Alexandrov. Published 2013 by Blackwell Publishing Ltd.